2·20·18

Every woman wants a perfect figure, but nobody's perfect! Everyone—including models and actresses—has some sort of figure flaw she wishes would "go away." Now Oleda Baker, well-known New York fashion model, offers an expert, thorough, systematic approach to a subject in which every woman has an instinctive interest.

In this highly individualized guide, Oleda and her sister, Francey Petty, tell how to highlight strong points and artfully conceal weak points, to take your figure that one (or two or three) steps further to a picture of total attractiveness. In more than 100 illustrated pages the magic of figure illusion comes alive.

You'll learn how to self-evaluate your figure, and the best way to deal with individual problems or any combination of them. You'll discover how to choose the right clothing for you: the proper styles, colors, fabrics, undergarments, sportswear, and accessories to enhance *your* figure. Find out how to balance your figure, dress and carry it effectively; how the proper clothing can shed pounds instantly; how to appear slimmer or curvier than you are. There is even a chapter on how *not* to give the illusion of an imperfect figure (in case you are one of the lucky ones with a great figure).

A complete encyclopedia of "Dos" and "Don'ts" for all kinds of trouble spots including legs, thighs, stomach, bust, buttocks, hips, waist, arms, chin—a lot of small expert tips that add up to a big important difference.

Now women from seventeen to seventy can stop fretting and guessing while learning *How to Create the Illusion of a More Perfect Figure.* Stop bemoaning the fact that you don't have the proportions of some mythical perfect somebody. And remember that an "illusion" that appears consistently and successfully may just not be an illusion, after all.

ALSO BY OLEDA BAKER

The Model's Way to Beauty, Slenderness, and Glowing Health
The I Hate to Make Up Book
29 Forever

HOW TO CREATE THE ILLUSION OF A MORE PERFECT FIGURE

Oleda Baker
and Francey Petty

Illustrated by Paul Hoover

PRENTICE-HALL, INC., Englewood Cliffs, New Jersey

How to Create the Illusion of a More Perfect Figure
by Oleda Baker and Francey Petty

Printed in the United States of America
Prentice-Hall International, Inc., London
Prentice-Hall of Australia, Pty. Ltd., Sydney
Prentice-Hall of Canada, Ltd., Toronto
Prentice-Hall of India Private Ltd., New Delhi
Prentice-Hall of Japan, Inc., Tokyo
Prentice-Hall of Southeast Asia Pte. Ltd., Singapore
Whitehall Books Limited, Wellington, New Zealand
10 9 8 7 6 5 4 3 2 1

Library of Congress Cataloging in Publication Data
Baker, Oleda.
How to create the illusion of a more perfect figure.
Includes index.
1. Clothing and dress. I. Petty, Francey, joint author. II. Title
TT507.B34 391'.07'2 77-22825
ISBN 0-13-404475-4

To women everywhere
mindful of one of womankind's constant creative endeavors
creating the illusion of a more perfect figure

Our thanks to:
Editor Carol Cartaino, who wouldn't let us do less than our best;
Vernice Gabriel, without whose help we couldn't have achieved it;
and our dedicated production editors, Shirley Stein and Ethel Waters.

INTRODUCTION

Nobody's perfect! Not even the most beautiful and attractive women—including models and actresses. Everyone has some kind of figure flaw to deal with—shoulders too narrow, hips too wide, neck too short, bust too small or large, for example—and most of us have more than one. But regardless of your figure problem, this book will tell you exactly how to deal with it—how to conceal your weak points, make the most of your strong points, and in general take your figure that one or two or three steps further toward creating a picture of *total* attractiveness.

You will find in these pages an individualized program for making the most of the figure you happen to have been born with. We'll show you how to do something about the things you've always secretly (or not so secretly) fretted about because "they're inherited—there's nothing I can do about them." As for the figure flaws you *can* do something about by the ordinary means—like losing those five or ten or twenty pounds you've been meaning to get rid of—the advice we're going to give you will enable you instantly and painlessly to enhance your body image while you are finally losing them.

You will learn the art of figure illusion—it can be learned. We've all done a little of it by trial and error. Actresses, models, and the "Beautiful People" have done it for years. Haven't you seen entertainers on TV that you knew had figure flaws but were so impressed with their general appearance that you thought they looked fantastic? What they have learned is simply how to achieve this illusion for their individual figure.

Remember that your appearance talks before you open your mouth. The success of your appearance depends first on your *knowing your figure flaws* and then dealing with them by camouflaging these drawbacks. Money is not the most important ingredient of a good appearance. It can buy expensive clothes—but not figure balance, not figure know-how, and not good taste.

The undeniable fact is that clothes—one of a woman's greatest allies in presenting herself as an alluring creature—are often responsible for creating precisely the opposite effect. Most women admit they are not sure of the best way to dress, but what to do about it is an unanswered question. There seems to be no way to obtain a basic education in the right clothes to buy, the hairstyle that looks best for each individual woman's face and body, the best accessories to complete her outfit. The rapid industrialization of the clothing industry in America has brought every fashion imaginable to the doorstep of all classes of citizens. Decisions have literally been "dumped" in the laps of today's women—and the majority can't cope. Before industry brought fashion to the masses, the well-to-do and elegant were *told* by their designers what looked best on them. Today, even the woman of limited means has a choice of every kind of fashion, and she has only her own opinion or her best friend, or husband, to assist her in the creation of her own particular style of disaster.

And it is a disaster! How do we know? By looking at women walking along Michigan Avenue in Chicago, Fifth Avenue in New York City, Collins Avenue in Miami Beach, and other fashionable streets (and a lot of "ordinary" streets) throughout our country. We have seen the oversized clogs or platforms in which our bewildered sister is stumbling, the gobs of jewelry all on at one time along with scarves and outlandish hairstyles, the clashing colors and designs poorly suited for her figure type: heavy-hipped women wearing gathered skirts, dresses with horizontal designs, the wrong style of pants with huge hip pockets stuffed with tissues; short women wearing middy skirts and oversize design prints. The list is long and horrible. On every hand is unisex clothing so successful that female identity is entirely lost. The well-to-do depend on Halston or Dior creations to give them "style"—even though nine times out of ten it's the wrong style for them.

In this book we'll provide charts and diagrams that will help you "map out" your own body image and pinpoint your personal figure problems (there may even be one you've never quite focused on—though it's affecting the appearance you present, every day of your life). We will then tell you exactly what to do to create the illusion of a more perfect figure. You will learn the all-important technique of balancing your body; in every situation, what to wear and how to wear it; how to choose the best undergarments and accessories; the types and colors of fabrics most flattering for you—a lot of small expert tips that add up to a big important difference: how to see yourself as a total picture instead of dressing in sections.

You will find that the ability and willingness to make the most of your figure and appearance will help you in a great many ways. Knowing that you look your best gives you confidence and helps you feel your best. As you improve your overall body image (and self-concept), you will find your entire life-style—home, work, family, children, social life—steadily improving in subtle ways.

You will notice that we have concerned ourselves with length, style, color, and so on, strictly in terms of what looks best for a particular figure type. This is because we firmly believe you must forget (or "gracefully ignore") fads and trends. The "optical illusion" of what looks best on you has far more impact, and clear-cut benefit, than what happens to be in at any given moment. Of course there are occasions, and situations, where wearing the immediately fashionable may be inescapable, but in general, the woman who follows her trained sense of what looks best on her serves herself better, and makes a more lasting impression on the people she meets, than if she wore the latest thing (which, of course, will change by tomorrow).

How to Create the Illusion of a More Perfect Figure is the first book of its kind: a thorough, systematic approach to a subject in which every woman has an instinctive interest; an encyclopedia of figure problems and how to solve them. It will teach you how to balance your figure even if you weigh 175 pounds; if you have the top of one person and the bottom of another. It will show you how to appear slimmer or curvier than you are by choosing the best styles, fabrics, colors, and accessories for YOU.

So it's time to stop guesswork; it's time to stop living with a feeling that you just don't measure up; it's time to stop letting clothing manufacturers or salespeople tell you what styles are "in" when they have no idea what your figure problems may be.

It's time to stop bemoaning the fact that you don't have the proportions of some mythical perfect classic somebody, and time to set about doing the things you can do to bring the body you have to as perfect a state as it can be, so that you present a convincing picture of allover attractiveness.

Paralyzed by the sight of someone else's perfect legs or bosom, you can sometimes forget the very assets that you yourself have. What we want to do is help you present them in the most effective way so that you can be sure of your share of "the action."

So find your figure or spot problems and start putting into practice the advice in these pages that will give *you* a more "perfect" figure than you ever dreamed you could have. "Naturally" perfect or calculatedly perfect? Who cares? Remember that an "illusion" that appears consistently and successfully may just not be an illusion, after all. . . . And the results that come to you will be very real indeed.

CONTENTS

Chapter One

LEARNING TO SEE YOURSELF AS OTHERS SEE YOU

Your appearance speaks before you say a word. It gives other people clues to your personality, social status, a hint as to your occupation, and even what you expect out of life. You have all heard the timeless expression, "First impressions are the most important." This adage has stayed around so long because it has proved to be true. As unfair as this may seem to people who like to emphasize the importance of inner beauty, we live in a world that dwells on—or at least takes into strong account—superficial, initial impressions. Francey and I are not here to judge the justice of our society; we are here to tell you how to get the most out of your appearance . . . and that's just what we intend to do! So let's deal with this fact of life realistically in order to stimulate people to want to know you better, well enough to know the "real you"!

NO MATTER HOW BEAUTIFUL ANY PART OF THE WHOLE IS, IT IS THE WHOLE THAT MUST LOOK BEAUTIFUL. The Germans even have a word for it: *Gestalt.* It means a "unified whole; a configuration, pattern, or organized field having . . . properties that cannot be derived from the summation of its component parts." The total image of a person is created by how all the individual facets of appearance all fit or work together—and by how a person shows her awareness of her total appearance in the form of poise, carriage, and posture. A woman can have expensive jewelry, an exquisite hairstyle, and the most up-to-date or chic clothing, and each element in itself could be striking, but they could be incongruous, disappointing, unflattering when put together as an outfit. Don't be guilty of throwing things together without giving yourself a good study in the mirror.

Getting yourself together properly is a very wise investment of time and money. People not only react to you differently, but your own feelings change about yourself; this gives you a feeling of self-confidence, which in turn influences still more subtly how others see you. To give you an example of people's reactions to different types of appearances, we would like to cite this episode: Francey and I dressed in a way that would have rated us about 40 in general appearance on a scale of 1 to 100. We were disguised to some degree in that our hair was tucked under scarves and caps and we were wearing sunglasses. We went into a department store that is known for its patient and well-trained sales personnel. The salesperson waited on us pleasantly; she did her job. In the afternoon, we went back to the same counter, same salesperson. Both times we made sure there was no other customer also waiting for the salesperson's attention. The second time we rated 90-95 on the scale. We were waited on with more personal feeling and the salesperson was more concerned with what we wanted. We were shown many more choices of items and were told "Thank you" and "Have a good day." Think for a moment. Haven't you noticed how even the momentary encounter with the toll taker or the UPS man (or your old boyfriend) becomes a more pleasant experience when you happen to be "together," than when you've been caught in your curlers and an old housedress?

Mr. Webster defines "general appearance" in the following way:

General—concerned with the main or overall features; lacking in detail; not specific.

Appearance—the look or outward impression of anything.

Your general appearance can be the deciding factor in obtaining that position you have been longing for; it can help you snare a lover or husband; it can help you maintain a marriage. Adversely, an ill-planned or unkempt image can certainly stand in the way of acquiring the things you want most in life. It is amazing how we seem to forget one of the most significant words from Webster's definition—the word *overall*—when we are trying to find ways to make ourselves look attractive and capture attention.

So how do we do it? There is a very simple rule: Dress first for a total look, then for detail.

Begin by consulting your best friend. No, not your girl friend; and not your diamonds, either—they're only your second-best friends. A FULL-LENGTH MIRROR is your truest confidante, especially if you make the proper use of it. Don't use a small mirror that only shows a kneecap at a time, but a full-length mirror that shows *everything*. If you will be honest with your mirror, it will be honest with you. "Face up" so that you can "cover up" is a long-term trick of many entertainers and models you think were perfect to begin with.

When you have put together your clothing, accessories, shoes, and hairstyle, it is only your full-length mirror that will tell you if you are a "unified whole." Models have learned through their work *never* to add even a necklace without looking at it in a mirror as part of their total dress.

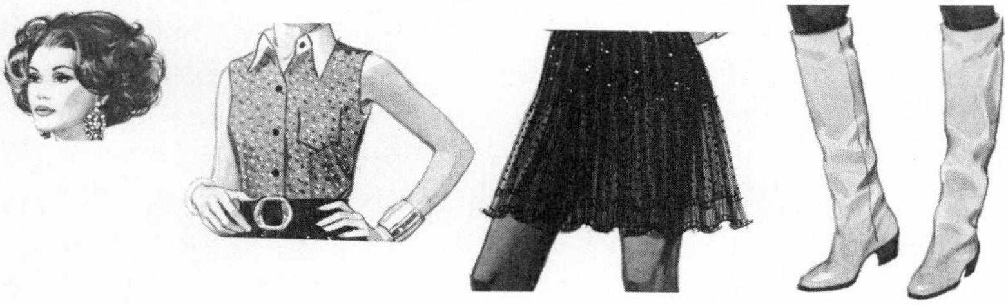

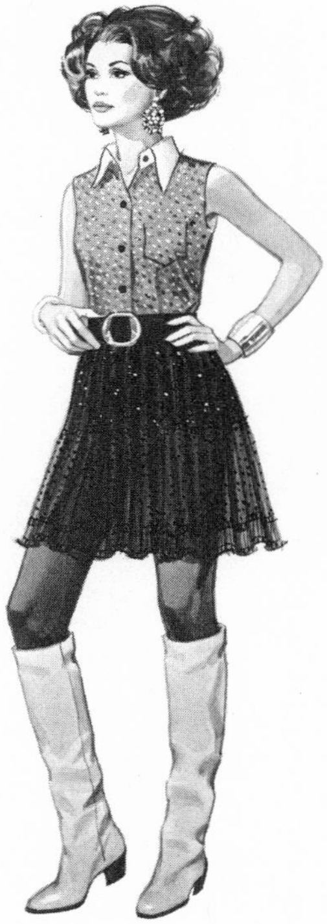

No matter how beautiful any one part is—it is the whole that must look beautiful. A woman can have expensive jewelry, an exquisite hairstyle, the most up-to-date or chic clothing, with each thing in itself being quite striking, but they could be incongruous and unflattering when put together as an outfit

When you are completely dressed, learn to look at yourself in the full-length mirror—standing five feet away from it. What *total* image do you give? Is your head or hair too large or small for the proportion of your body? Would it be better if your clothing hugged your hips a little more to balance with your shoulders? Do you have too many accessories? If you are not sure—remove some of them. Do the colors go well together? Does the outfit play down your negative points and play up your assets? Are your clothes the right length—including your sleeve length? If your answer to all of these questions is not positive, then you are not ready to present your image to the world.

Learning to criticize yourself at home is no different from the criticizing of another woman's appearance in public that we do all the time. But it *is* harder to be *objective* about ourselves.

To take an honest look at your silhouette, stand five feet away from the mirror with no lights coming from the front, but

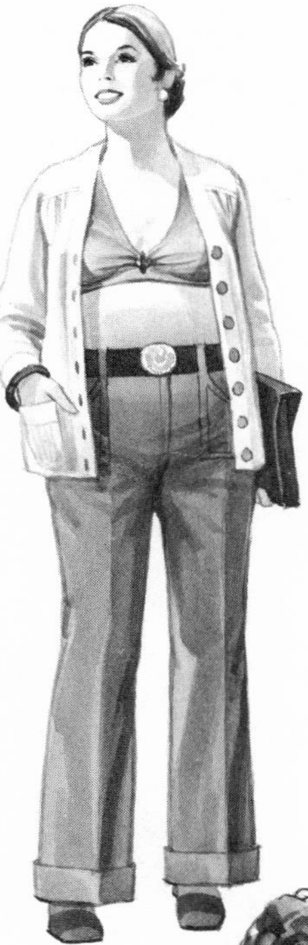

a strong light in back of you. You will see the same silhouette that other people see of you. It's a good test—try it! A HAND MIRROR is a must to see what image you give from the back and side or "profile" views. It's what everyone else sees, so don't ignore it. Use the hand mirror not only in this test, but at *all* times to check body views. If you are used to checking your full-face view and leaving it at that, you may discover unsuspected problems or defects in your rear or side view that must be dealt with. Remember that *these* are the images of you that everyone else sees *all the time.*

Once you have checked a particular outfit on yourself, it's only necessary the next time to check yourself in the mirror for details. While looking yourself over, make sure hooks and snaps are closed. Check for runs in your stockings. Is a hem out? Is any part of your outfit torn, wrinkled, or spotted?

Ask your mirror to be very critical and tell you when you are not "the fairest one of all." When it tells you "Not today," then do something *instantly* about it. Don't answer back by saying: "I'll do better tomorrow." You will make an impression today and it had better be your best. You never know what excitement is waiting for you the rest of the day. Now, if you say, "Oh, nothing will happen today, it never does; I'll wait for a special occasion to get myself together," well, no wonder nothing ever happens! The horse comes before the cart. You get yourself together so something *will* happen!

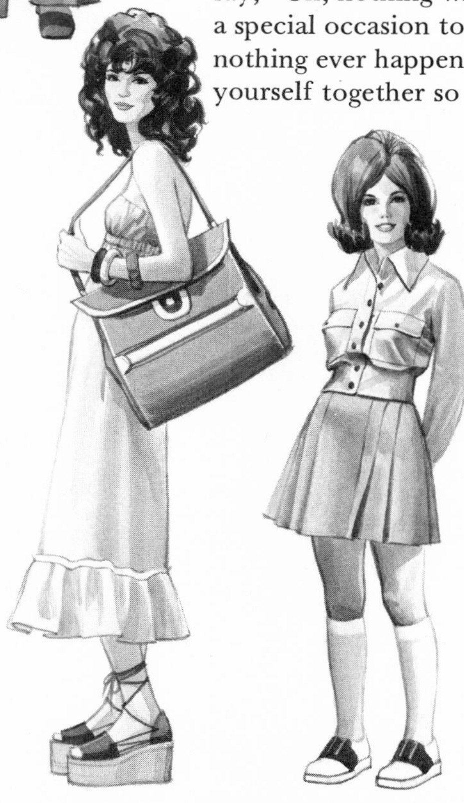

We must learn to look at the total image that we present, to see ourselves in full view, as we do others (and as others do us)

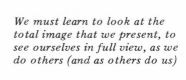

Chapter Two

AN HONEST LOOK AT YOUR PROPORTIONS

Before you can hope to present your figure at its best you must take an honest look at it, getting to know the problems and the potentials of your own image or silhouette. When you complete this chapter, there will be no doubt as to what they are. Once you know them, then and only then can you do something about them. You will be ready to move on to the positive changes that you can make.

We are always "mentally" improving our figure in a multitude of ways, but the fact is that certain aspects of it are unchangeable—things such as height, bone structure, and basic figure proportions.

You *can* make improvements, such as losing weight, and improving overall body tone, or gaining weight if you are underweight. There are spot exercise programs to reduce or add to certain parts of the body. (And there are a host of books, magazine articles, and courses to help you do these things, including Oleda's *Model's Way to Beauty, Slenderness, and Glowing Health.*)

But you may have tried (and even succeeded in sticking with) most of the standard self-improvement paths and discovered that they do not necessarily bring you all the way to the perfect figure, the ideal proportions, you've pictured in your mind. This is because you are still always working with certain "unchangeable" aspects of that figure you were born with; and because there are visual rules you must learn—and will, in the course of this book—that will always strongly affect how other people see your figure.

First take the measurements of each part of your body listed and fill in the blanks. Measurements should be taken with your usual bra and panties donned, since the measurements are taken for the preparation of your figure balance when it is dressed. While you are standing in only your bra and panties, measure yourself with a flexible measuring tape, holding it snugly, but not tightly, around the nine key areas listed below.

1. neck ________
2. upper arm ________
3. bust ________
4. waist ________
5. hips ________
6. upper thigh ________
7. mid-thigh ________
8. calf ________
9. ankle ________

How to Measure Each Part

Neck—Place the tape around the middle of the neck.

Upper arm—Place the tape four inches down from the armpit.

Bust—Place the tape over the fullest part of the bust and straight across the back.

Waist—Measure your natural waistline, the smallest part. Don't hold your breath in.

Hips—Measure the fullest part, usually about seven inches below the natural waistline on short figures, nine inches below on tall ones.

Upper thigh—Place the tape as high as possible and pull it straight around your leg.

Mid-thigh—Measure halfway between the upper thigh and the knee.

Calf—Measure around the largest part of the calf.

Ankle—Place tape around the smallest part, just above the anklebone.

Next, take these measurements and fill them in lightly with pencil on one of the appropriate height and weight charts. (You may make a mistake or wish to change the chart if your figure should change a few months from now.) Choose one of the three charts, according to your height. If you are short (5′4″ or below), fill out the column marked "short." If you are average height (5′4″ to 5′7″), fill out the "medium" column. If you are tall (5′7″ or over) fill out the "tall" column.

A simple way to determine your bone structure ("frame")

size is to measure your wrist. Take the measurement at the point of the "bump" on your wrist. Measure *both* wrists. If wrists are different, add the total and divide by 2. If you have broken one wrist, use the unbroken one. For women a wrist measurement under 6 inches means a small bone frame; between 6-6½ inches means a medium frame; over 6½ inches—large.

Judge the proportioning of your figure as follows. For example, in a woman with a medium frame, who is 5′7″ and weighs 125 pounds, if her wrist measures 6 inches, her ankle should be 1½ times the wrist; her calf should be twice the size of her wrist; her thigh, 3 times the size; her waist, 4 times the size; and her hips and bust, 6 times the size of her wrist. If your measurements fall within a 3-inch range in certain spots, your body is still well proportioned. Given a 6-inch wrist, the range of measurement for a perfectly proportioned figure would be ankle 8-10, calf 11-13, mid-thigh 17-19, waist 23-26, hip 35-38, bust 34-37. Generally speaking, measurements of your bust (with bra on) and your hips should be the same (hips can be an inch or two larger) for perfect proportions, and your waist should be 10 inches smaller.

A simple way to tell if you are overweight, if scales scare you, is to subtract your waist measurement from your height in inches, without shoes, and if the result is 36 or greater, you are not too heavy—that is, 5′7″ converted to inches = 67. Subtract 24-inch waist = 43 inches. Since 43 is higher than 36, the woman is not overweight. (This won't apply to pregnant women or to professional athletes, who carry a lot of extra muscle.)

Don't forget that the length of the various parts of your body also plays an important role in the picture you present. On a person of perfect proportions, the distance from the pelvic bone to the bottom of the feet, standing, should be equal to the distance from the top of the head to the pelvic bone. A perfectly proportioned body would be 7½ to 8 times the length of the head (measured from the top of the head to the chin).

If the measurement from the pelvic bone down to the feet is 1½ inches or more shorter than the top measurement, you are probably short-legged.

A simple test for short-waistedness is the length of the arms. Hang your arms down at your side by your thighs. If your *wrist bone* bypasses your coccyx bone (that is your tail bone, which is the last vertebra on your spine) by more than 1½ inches, you are probably short-waisted and must compensate.

HEIGHT AND WEIGHT CHART

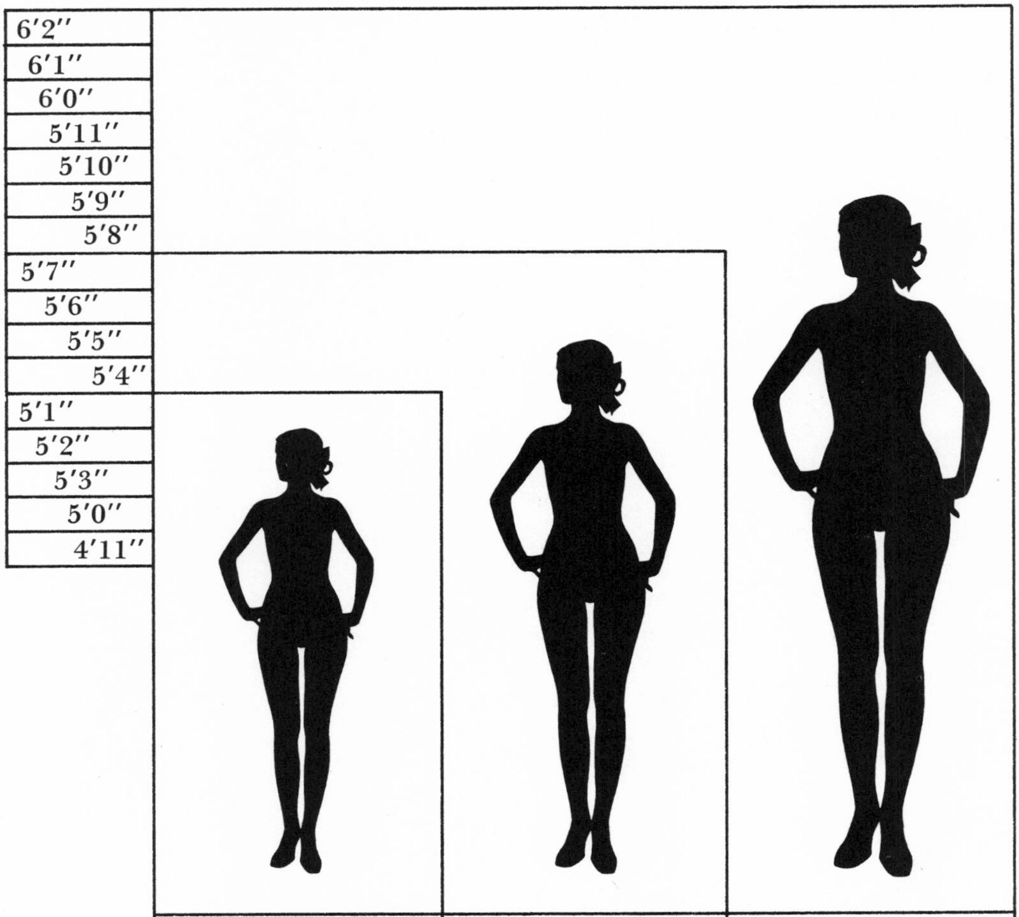

	SHORT			MEDIUM			TALL		
	Thin	Average	Heavy	Thin	Average	Heavy	Thin	Average	Heavy
Small frame									
Medium frame									
Large frame									

This chart will help you identify your figure type. You will need this information for other parts of this book

FACING UP SO YOU CAN COVER UP

As we have said earlier, it is not enough to know your height, weight, and even the measurements of every part of your body. You must see your total image in proportion before this book can be of real service to you. (Yes, it is possible to live with yourself for years, even decades, and spend endless hours looking in the mirror, and never take a clear analytic look at your total figure.)

The easiest thing is to have a friend take a Polaroid (black and white might be best) shot of you, wearing bra and panties and your usual hairdo, from the front and back, and also from the side. Be sure she takes the picture close enough so that you "fill the frame" of the picture. Then, with a pen or marker, outline your *silhouette* only.

With a piece of tracing paper, pick up the silhouette only and you will have before you a stark, simple picture of your outline or overall image, from each side, without all the details and features that usually distract from this essential fact.

Having the side as well as front and back views will graphically point out that measurements alone do not tell the story—each figure has individual differences of width versus depth of various parts of the body, that are part of the image we create, part of what adds or detracts from our appearance.

If you have an artistic bent, you could try taking the measurements (width and length) of various parts of your body and "plotting" them on a piece of large-scale graph paper. Now you will have the "outline" of your own body. After studying it closely, we can start balancing it by deciding on the best style of clothing for you.

For example, if your silhouette looks like this, it's obvious that your hips are larger than your shoulders. So two major sections to consult would be "Hips Too Large" and "Shoulders Too Narrow."

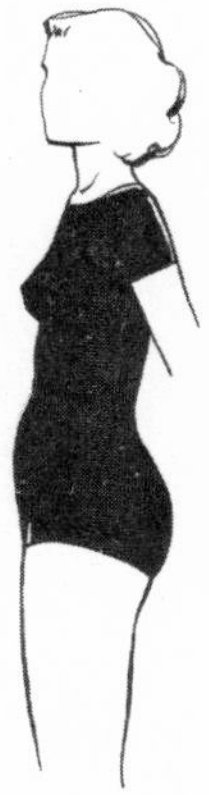

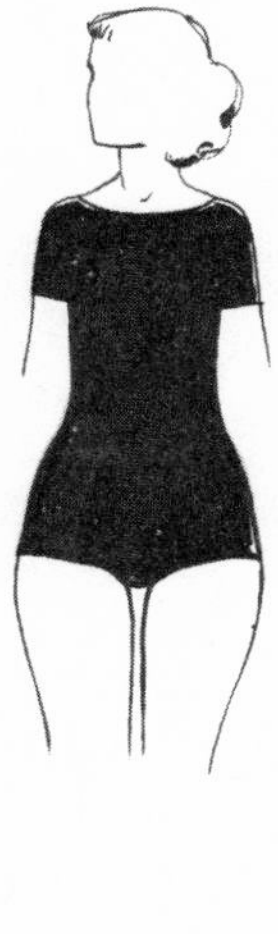

Don't forget there's more than one side to the story

After reading both of these sections you would find out how to make your hips look narrow by choice of skirt and how to broaden your shoulders so your hips would look less out of proportion.

As you read on, you will find more ways to pinpoint your problems and correct them to give the illusion of a more perfect figure. You will learn how to choose and wear everything correctly, from hairdo through every type of clothing, to jewelry and shoes. So make your decision right now to complete each phase of this project to become the YOU you want to be.

Chapter Three

SPOT PROBLEMS

Would you believe that even Raquel Welch has spot figure problems? They are minor ones, but in her business she must appear perfect. She has achieved this perfection by wearing the proper clothing to de-emphasize her trouble spots. Models, whose careers depend on their "perfect" figures, by no means have perfect figures! Some have legs too long or too short for their bodies; some have heads too small for their bodies; some have narrow shoulders; others have bosoms too large or too small—but they all look beautiful and most appear nearly perfect. They have learned from long studies of the mirror and their own photos what their spot problems are and how to disguise them.

Francey and I are very much included when it comes to having spot figure problems, of course. (I have more spot problems than my sister.) Now you may say, "It doesn't appear that way to me," and that is exactly our point. There are times when it is a virtue to be deceiving!

So let's go step by step—find your spot problems and go to it! (The following Spot Problem discussions have been arranged in alphabetical order.)

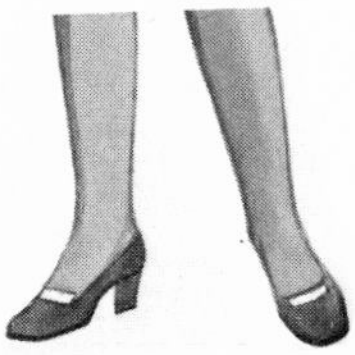

Do Wear

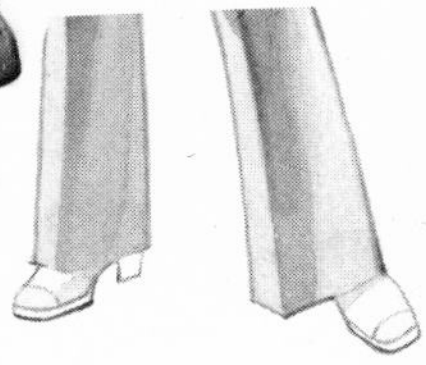

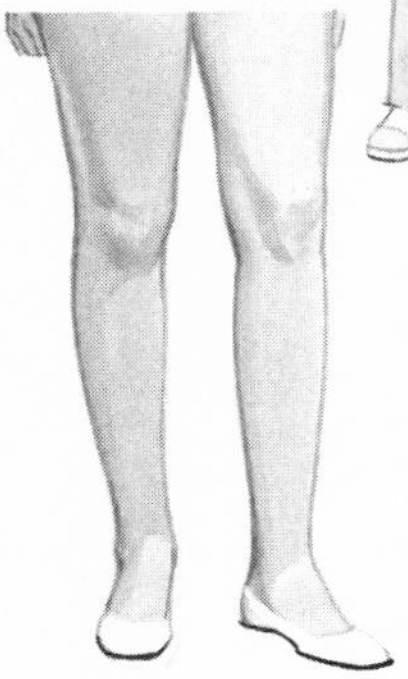

Avoid

ANKLES

Too Thick

DO WEAR:

a. slacks if you have an exceptional problem and want to look your best
b. darker tone stockings—this does not mean you must wear very dark stockings; just medium-to-dark natural tones in whatever shade you select
c. substantial-looking shoes rather than a very small string or strap shoe
d. ankle-strap shoes if you must wear a strap shoe

AVOID:

a. long dresses and slacks which hit just above or in the middle of the ankles
b. light-color stockings and shoes
c. dainty or flat-heeled shoes
d. novelty colors and patterns in stockings and tights

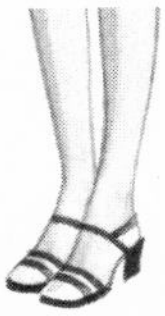

Do Wear

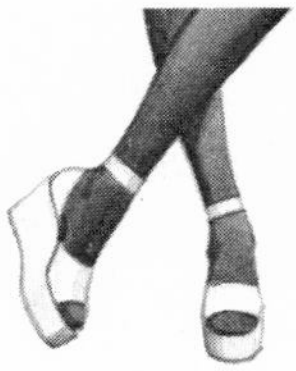

Avoid

Too Thin

DO WEAR:

a. medium- to light-tone stockings
b. delicate and lightweight shoes
c. thin-strap shoes

AVOID:

a. dark stockings
b. heavy clunky shoes
c. ankle-strap shoes

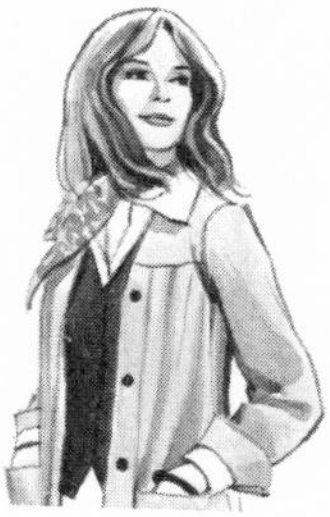

Do Wear

ARMS

Too Thin

DO WEAR:

a. long sleeves, preferably that cover the wrist all the way to the beginning of the hand
b. draped sleeves (not too full)
c. wide cuffs
d. if you must wear sleeveless, wear narrow strap over shoulder
e. delicate bracelet that is not too big for your wrist

AVOID:

a. halter-style tops
b. sleeveless garments that stop at end of shoulder
c. short, tight sleeves
d. puff sleeves
e. tight-fitting, clingy sleeve of any length
f. bulky bracelets

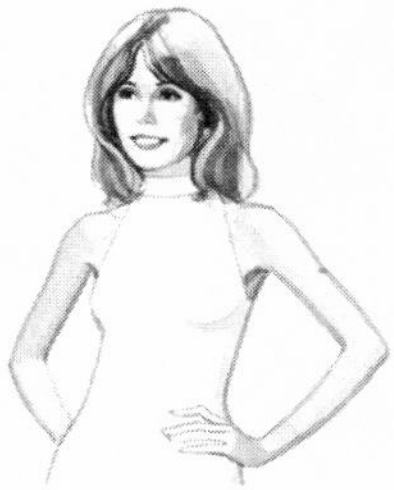

Avoid

Too Heavy

DO WEAR:

a. lightweight, close-fitting fabrics (not too tight)
b. well-cut sleeves, wide armholes, 3/4-length sleeves or reaching just above elbows
c. softly draped sleeves
d. stole or scarf draped over shoulders and arms
e. bulky bracelets

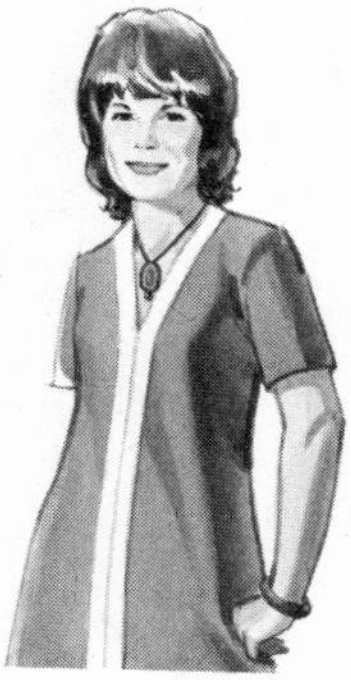

Do Wear

AVOID:

a. sleeveless garments
b. off-shoulder or strapless styles
c. short-sleeved garments
d. tight sleeves
e. delicate jewelry on the arms

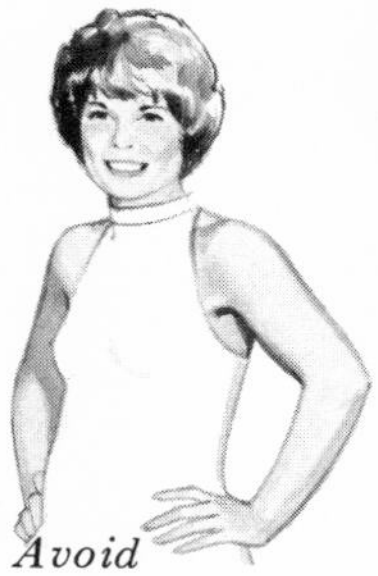

Avoid

Too Short

DO WEAR:

a. long sleeves, ¼ to ½ inch longer than the average person would
b. sleeves that are not too full (form-fitting is good if you have arms that are not too heavy)
c. sleeveless styles
d. long fingernails; it can give you a longer-looking arm. Paint them a medium-to-light color

AVOID:

a. short sleeves
b. full sleeves or layered sleeves
c. jewelry on arms (this cuts length of arm—wear a neck watch on a chain)
d. lots of rings

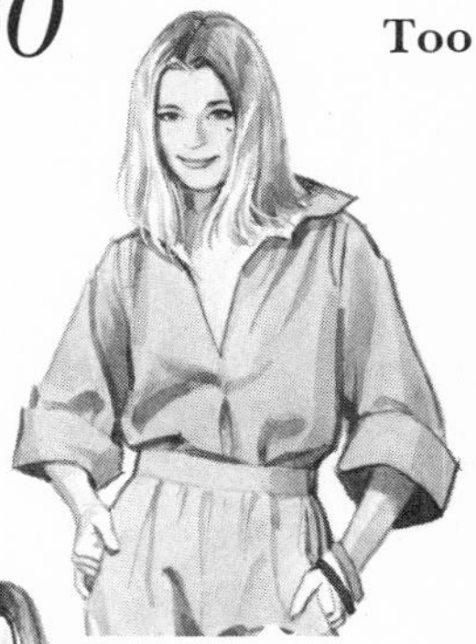

Do Wear

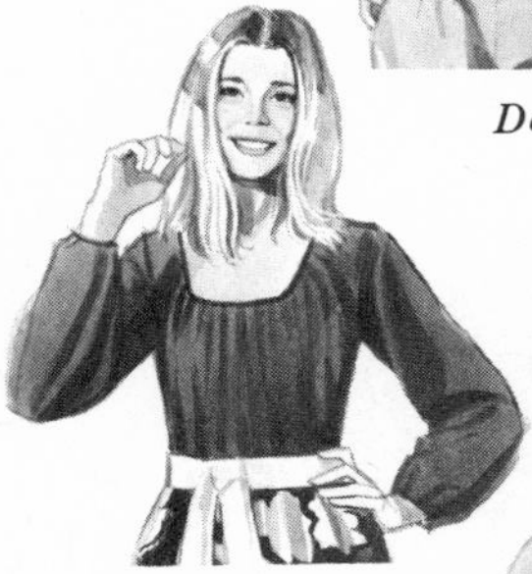

Avoid

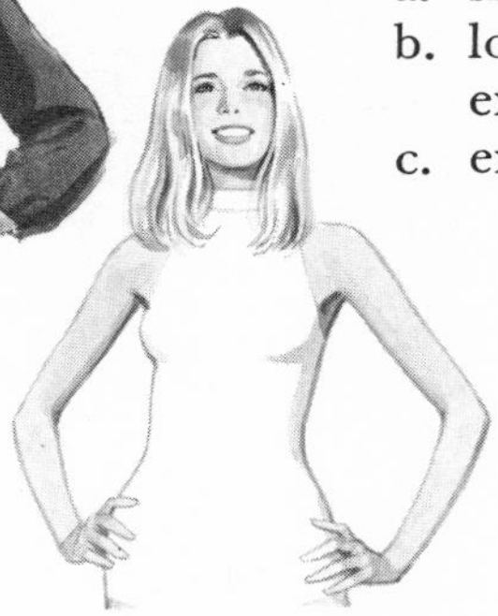

Too Long

DO WEAR:

a. short and 3/4-length sleeves
b. long sleeves that do not extend past wrist or long sleeves that are ¼ to ½ inch shorter than your normal length
c. full sleeves
d. layers if the weather permits
e. cuffed sleeves (they cut length of arm)
f. bracelets and rings—they give the illusion of a shorter arm

AVOID:

a. sleeveless styles
b. long sleeves that are too short—the problem is only exaggerated
c. exceptionally long fingernails

BACK

Too Wide

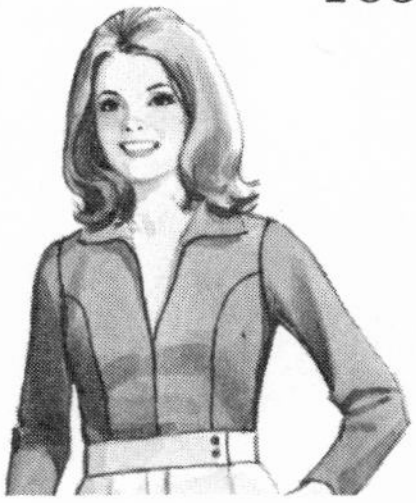

Do Wear

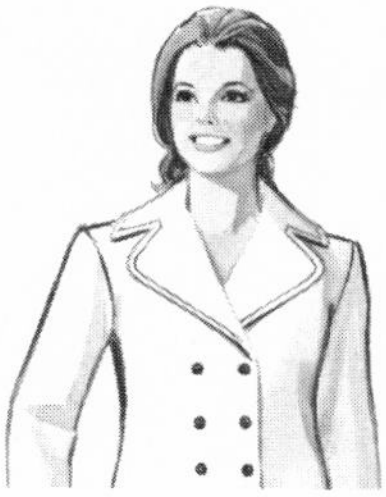

Avoid

DO WEAR:

a. closely fitted upper garments with vertical seams set in from each side
b. fabrics with vertical designs as much as possible
c. V-backs when possible
d. thicker straps, in shoulder-strap-style garments
e. hair past the shoulders if possible

AVOID:

a. horizontal lines in garment design and fabric design
b. bulky, loose blouses and tops
c. sweaters and tops that are too tight and clingy
d. shoulder pads
e. "spaghetti" or "string" straps (if you must wear shoulder-strap-type garments)
f. any sleeve that is not tailored

Too Narrow

DO WEAR:

a. clothing from the waist up that does not fit too tightly
b. the layered look
c. horizontal garment designs and fabric designs
d. blouses and jackets with slightly puffy sleeves at seam of sleeve and shoulder

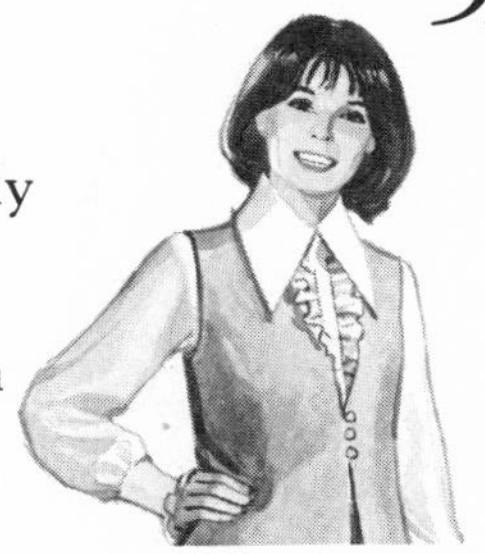

Do Wear

AVOID:

a. tight dark clothing above the waist
b. sleeveless styles
c. vertical lines on upper garments
d. belts that are too wide; they only emphasize a narrow back

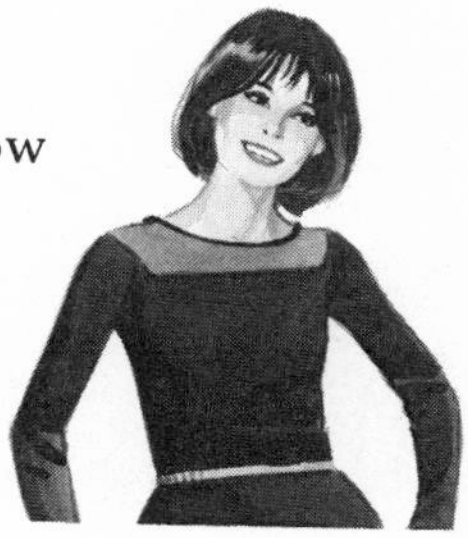

Avoid

Swayback (exaggerated curve in lower back)

The easiest way to check for swayback is to stand up against a wall with the back of your heels and the back of your head flush against the wall. If your back has the proper curve, you should be able to feel a space the width of two fingers between your back and the wall, right below the waistline. (Swayback that is strictly a posture defect can be corrected—see any good posture guide.)

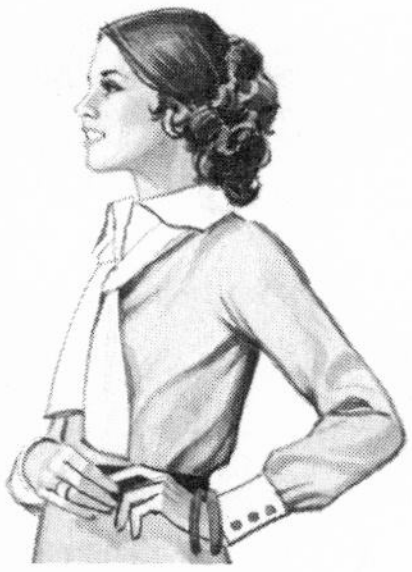

Do Wear

DO WEAR:

a. A-line dresses
b. shirtwaist-type dresses with thin belts
c. jackets or loose overlay clothing such as boleros and vests
d. loosely fitted clothing from your mid-back to below your waist

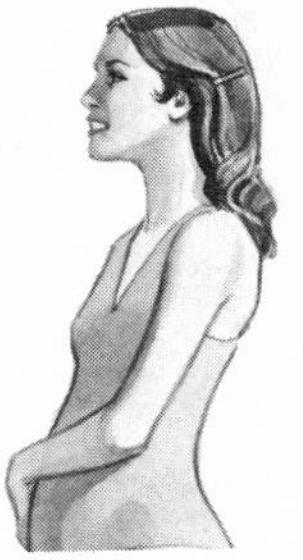

Avoid

AVOID:

a. clingy fabric from waist up
b. snugly-fitted clothing in the back
c. large belts

BUST

Too Large

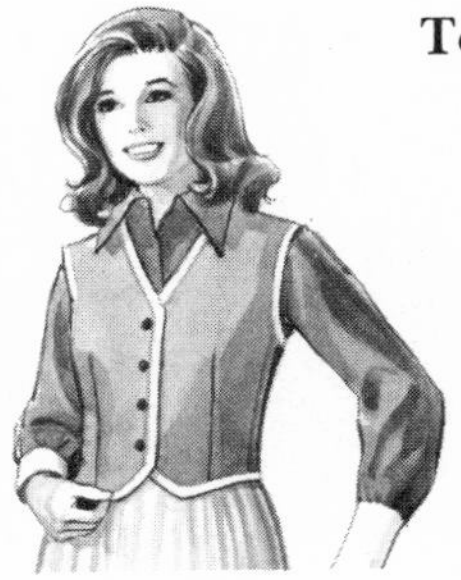

Do Wear

DO WEAR:

a. the correct bra (see Undergarments, Chapter Seven)
b. tops designed with simplicity; in particular, vertically designed tops (also vertical fabric designs)
c. oval, V-, and square necklines
d. soft lines, medium- to lightweight fabrics; these fabrics have an easy flow effect
e. dark bodices, contrasted with light bottom garments if you are not short or heavy-hipped

AVOID:

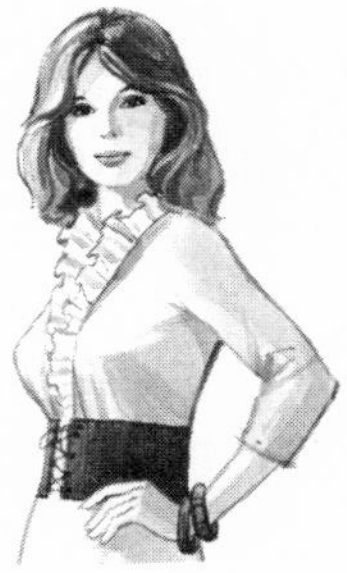

Avoid

a. fussy necklines
b. jewelry or scarves at bustline (see Accessories, Chapter Eight)
c. gathers, eye-catching trim, shirring, pleats or pockets at bustline
d. very tight upper garments
e. puffed or cap sleeves
f. double-breasted styles
g. wide belts
h. horizontal lines above the waist
i. tight skirts and slacks
j. big designs and flashy colors

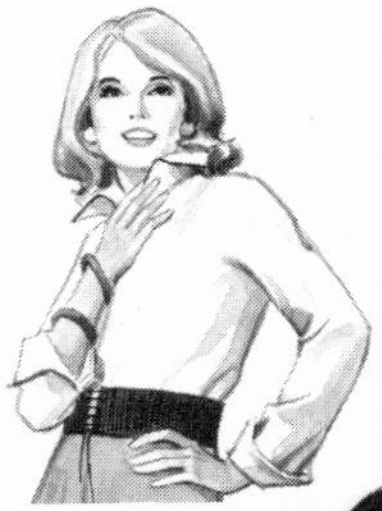

Too Small

Do Wear

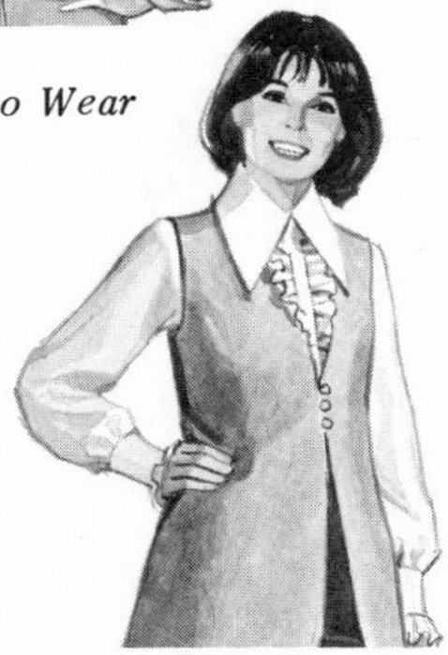

DO WEAR:

a. a bra especially designed for a small bosom (see Undergarments, Chapter Seven)
b. clothes that are loose, but not baggy—baggy clothing only makes one appear smaller
c. fussy tops if that's your style (easy gathers, tucks, bows, ruffled fronts, shirring, trim)
d. horizontal lines on top
e. double-breasted jackets
f. vests, boleros, the layered look on top
g. waist-cinching styles and designs (if you are not heavy-hipped)
h. peasant-style tops

AVOID:

a. very tight upper garments
b. vertical lines on top
c. tops that are too plain
d. sweaters or other extremely clingy upper garments
e. highly revealing tops

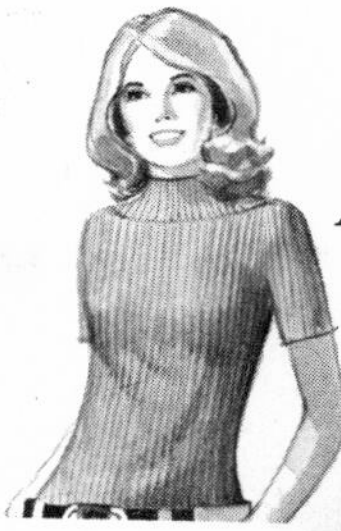

Avoid

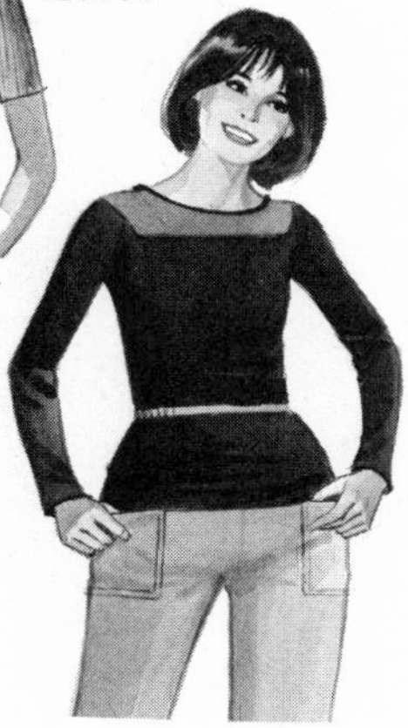

On the Small Side (wish to enhance)

The woman whose bust is on the "light medium" to small side, who would like to create a curvier effect, can profit from a somewhat different strategy than that outlined for *Bust Too Small.* (She is not so much trying to conceal a problem area as she is trying to enhance the effect of a modest, but attractive bosom.)

DO WEAR:

a. contour and push-up bras
b. form-fitting top garments (not *too* tight) chosen to highlight the curves that you do have—experiment trying on "clingy" and soft-fabric tops in a store till you find one that hugs just right
c. styles of dresses, swimsuits, and so on, in which the bust-band area is distinctly shaped or defined—this will help lend fullness
d. modestly low-cut garments
e. blouses and other tops a half size or full size smaller than you would normally wear (as long as the total look is not distorted or "too tight")
f. tops and bust-bands that are trimmed, gathered, ruffled, shirred, decorated at the bust, etc.
g. if you have an attractive upper chest, V necks, scoop necks, etc.
h. bonded-fabric tops
i. peasant-style tops
j. raglan sleeves

AVOID:

a. tops that are loose and "boxy"
b. very bulky fabrics or styles
c. extremely revealing or extremely low-cut styles

BUTTOCKS

Too Flat

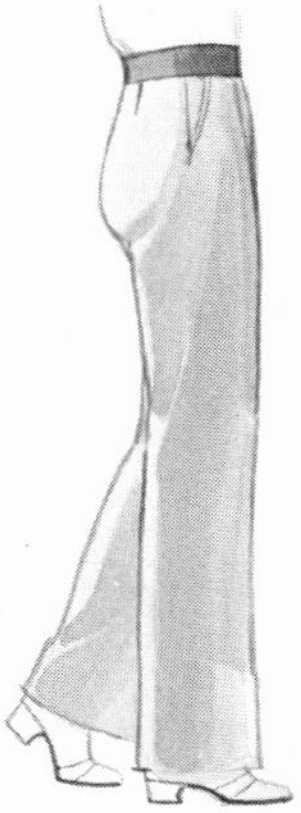

Do Wear

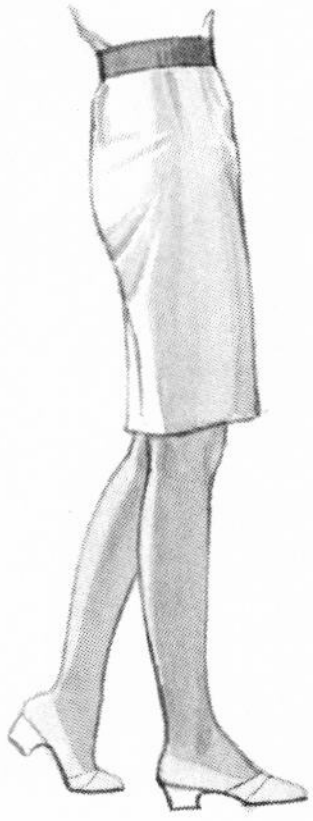

Avoid

DO WEAR:

a. a special undergarment (see Chapter Seven) if you have a severe problem
b. jackets or other tops which fall loosely down to the hip line (this actually "covers up" the problem)
c. belts and waistlines to make your waist appear as small as possible in order to make your derriere look as though it is more shapely
d. soft lines in the back (gathered or pleated skirts or dresses) made of soft, medium-weight fabric
e. skirts and slacks with well-tailored darts just below the waistline—nipping in at this area can make your derriere seem more rounded

AVOID:

a. fullness between waist and mid-buttock in a slim skirt or slacks—this calls attention to your problem
b. garments that fit too tightly at the widest point of the derriere—they make you look flatter

To Avoid Blending Into Legs

DO WEAR:

a. a light, well-fitted panty girdle if the garment calls for it (see Chapter Seven)
b. form-fitting garments a little looser than normal
c. A-line dresses and skirts
d. slacks that are slightly full

AVOID:

a. tight-fitting or clingy clothes in this problem area

Too Wide and Too Large

DO WEAR:

a. overblouses and jackets that extend to hip area (not bulky or full or baggy, though)
b. soft-flowing fabrics
c. A-line skirts and dresses, princess styles

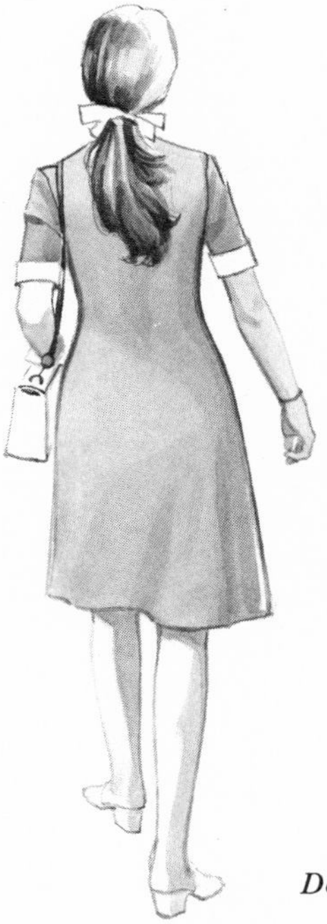

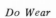

Do Wear

d. vertical designs or patterns toward front center of garment (this brings the attention away from the problem area)
e. dark-toned skirts, dresses, or slacks

AVOID:

a. tight waistbands
b. gathered-at-the-waist styles
c. wide belts
d. skirts and dresses that are too straight-line
e. very short or very full skirts
f. overlarge fabric designs
g. horizontal designs in fabric or garment
h. light-colored skirts or slacks
i. patch pockets near buttocks
j. shorts or slacks, when possible

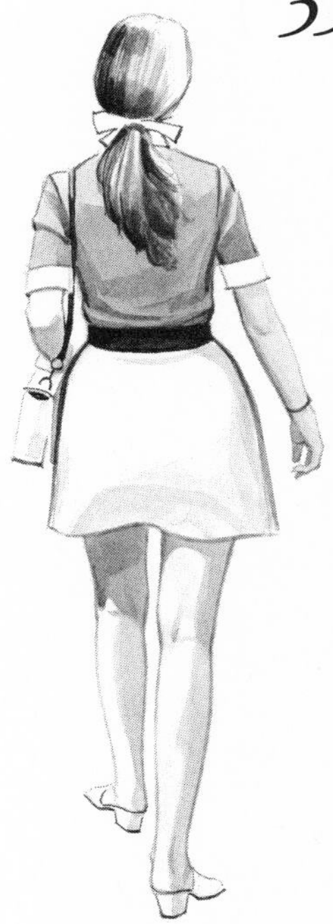

Avoid

CALVES

Too Thick

DO WEAR:

a. dress length at your knee or just above the smallest part of calf
b. full-cut leg styles of slacks
c. Bermuda shorts, rather than shorter styles
d. if you wear knickers, pedal pushers, or gauchos, choose styles with a fuller leg, rather than form-fitting (and the length should be at least 2 inches below the knee)
e. medium-to-dark shades of stockings, panty-hose, etc.
f. high heels, when possible

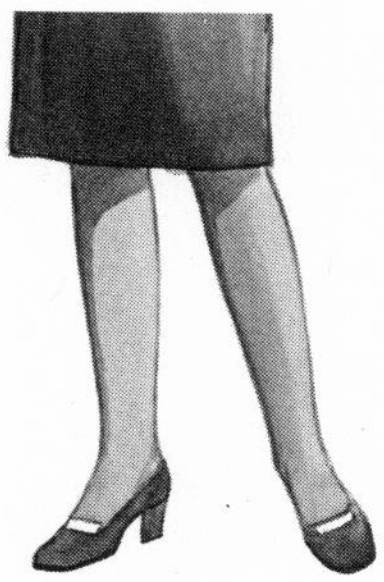

Do Wear

AVOID:

a. clothing hitting exactly at the largest point of your calf
b. tight slacks
c. short shorts, very short dresses, skirts
d. light-colored or patterned stockings, panty-hose, tights, etc.
e. knee socks, anklets (especially cuffed)
f. shoes that are too delicate-looking (or too heavy and massive-looking)
g. light-colored shoes, boots, etc.

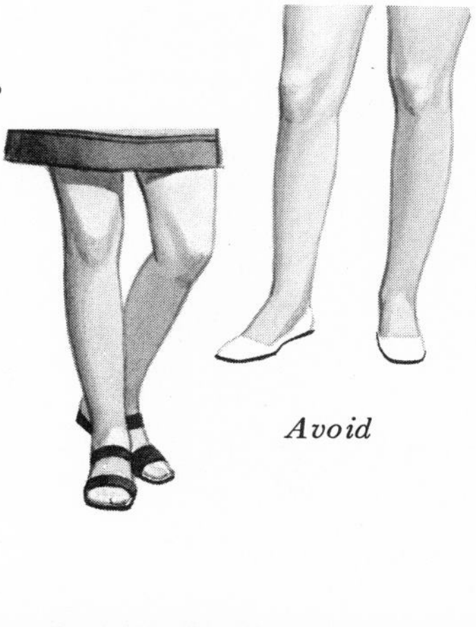

Avoid

Too Thin or No Curve

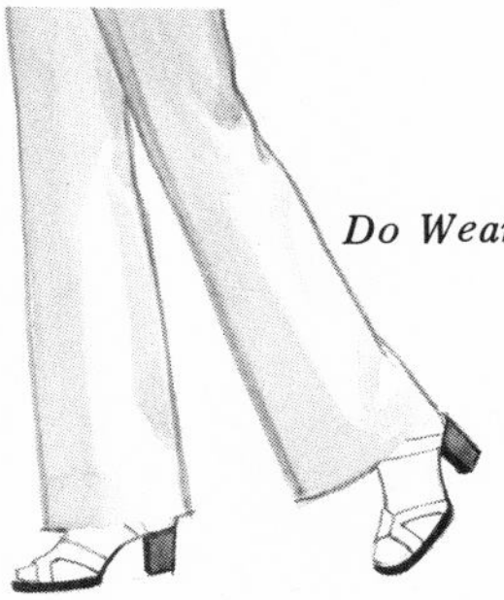

Do Wear

DO WEAR:

a. dresses and skirts of medium- to lightweight fabric which fall delicately to your calf
b. dress length just at the largest point of your calf
c. full-cut leg style slacks
d. pedal pushers, knickers, culottes, gauchos, and so on, that come almost to the fullest part of the calf
e. medium- to light-colored stockings (tights can soften the look of thin legs)
f. simple, graceful open shoes

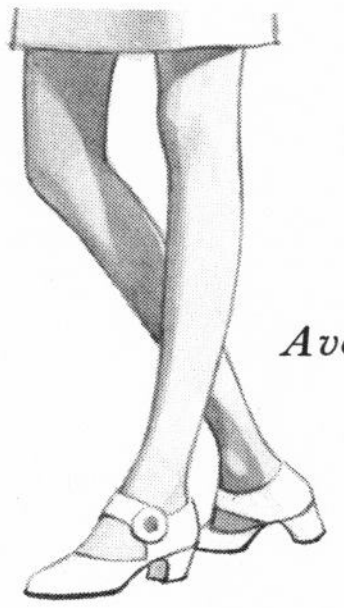

Avoid

AVOID:

a. extremely full skirts (unless they are floor length); the fuller the skirt, the smaller the legs appear
b. short shorts, very short skirts and dresses
c. shoes that are clumsy, heavy, or awkward-looking; they make legs appear even smaller
d. dark stockings or panty-hose

CHEST

Bony

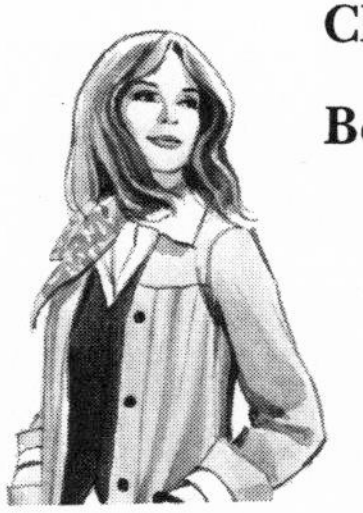

Do Wear

DO WEAR:

a. if you have long hair, wear it in a soft style that falls over the front of the shoulders
b. high necklines
c. scarves or opera-length necklaces
d. fussy necklines, such as big bows, ornate collars, ruffles
e. the layered look

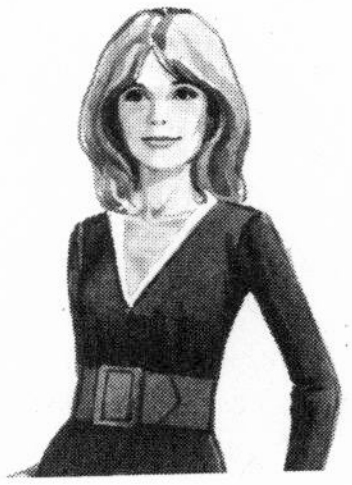

Avoid

AVOID:

a. deep-cut necklines, unless jewelry, scarf, or some other such accessory is worn

Wide

(A wide chest is one in which the basic width of the rib cage creates a figure wider at the chest than the hips—this does not always mean a full bust)

DO WEAR:

a. well-tailored blouses; the more fabric you "take away" on the sides, the slimmer you appear
b. fitted halter-style tops
c. shoulder-strap style garments (but not thin straps), to help cut the width
d. sleeveless-style garments that extend as far in toward the chest as possible
e. garments with vertical seams set in from each side
f. dark upper garments
g. vertical fabric and garment designs (even such things as contrasting-color vertical trim on upper garments)

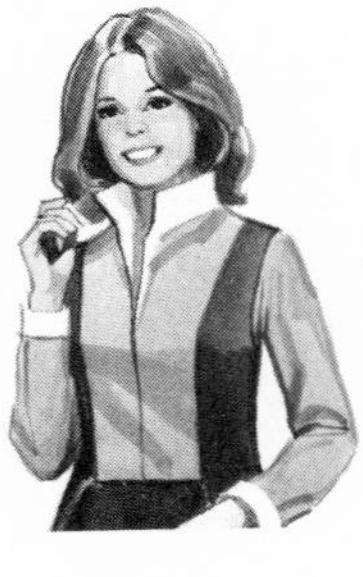

Do Wear

AVOID:

a. horizontal garment and fabric design
b. full blouses or sweaters
c. fabrics that are overly bulky
d. gathers on sides of blouse; always tuck gathers to each side of the front
e. sleeves that are gathered or puffed at shoulder
f. wide belts

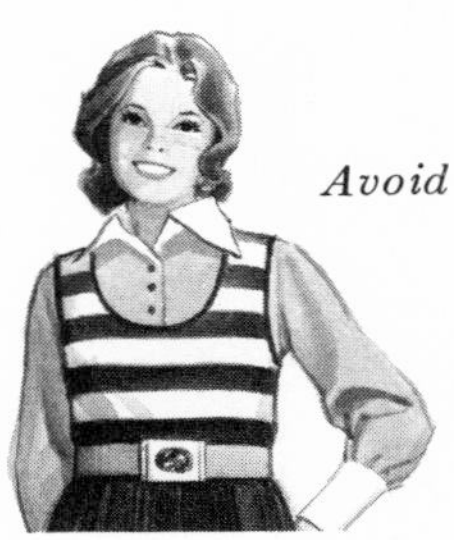

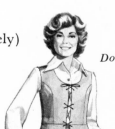

Avoid

Narrow

DO WEAR:

a. soft look on the top (let fabric lie over your chest loosely)
b. thin-strap shoulder-strap styles
c. full sleeves—they can give the illusion of a wider chest
d. vests, boleros, or other "layered look" clothing
e. horizontal garment designs and fabric designs
f. bulky fabrics when weather permits

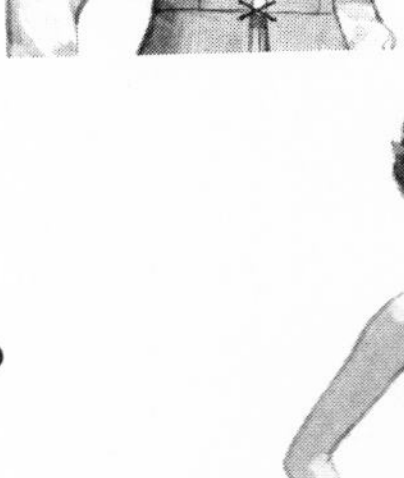

Do Wear

AVOID:

a. sleeveless and halter styles
b. very tight clothing across chest
c. vertical lines in clothing
d. black or very dark colors as much as possible on the top (unless full and loose)

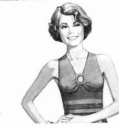

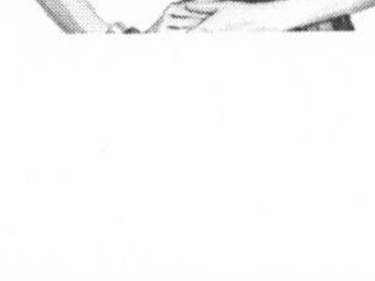

Avoid

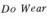

ELBOWS

Bony

If an elbow is bony, the arm is usually thin (see also our suggestions under "Arms Too Thin").

DO WEAR:

a. full-length sleeves or sleeves just past the elbow
b. very thin shoulder-strap styles, if you must wear something sleeveless (the thin strap can give the illusion of a fuller arm)

AVOID:

a. short puff sleeves
b. sleeve lengths falling between shoulder and elbow

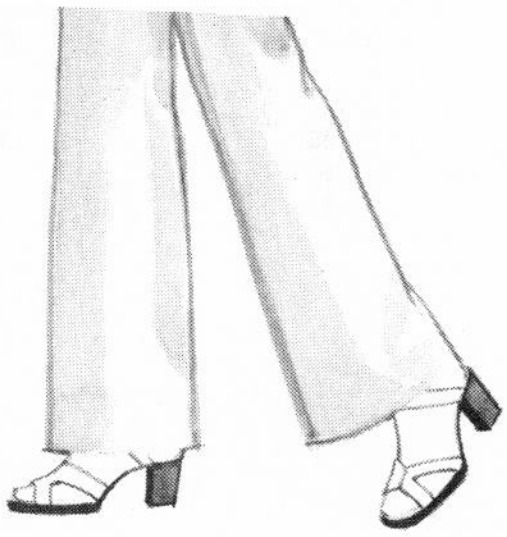

Do Wear

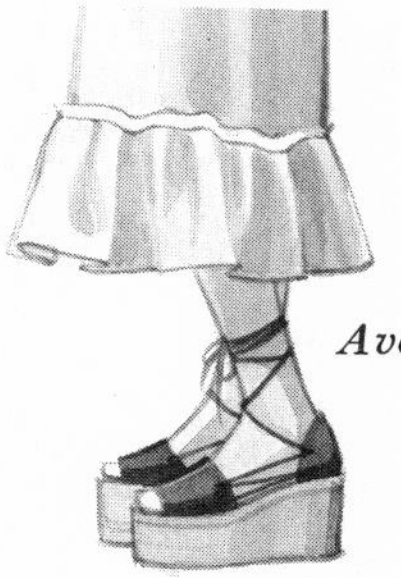

Avoid

FEET

Too Large

DO WEAR:

a. strap shoes and sandals (straps not too narrow)
b. simple delicate lines
c. low-cut shoes
d. open-toe and open-back shoes
e. a higher heel, when possible (if you are not too tall)

AVOID:

a. heavy, cumbersome shoes and boots
b. high-top shoes
c. shoes with too much ornamentation
d. light- to medium-colored shoes
e. flat-heeled shoes, when possible
f. very thick heeled or soled shoes
g. the pointed-toe look

HANDS

Too Large

DO WEAR:

a. long sleeves, not tight or full at the bottom
b. long sleeves with a ruffle around the edge (if you have exceptionally large hands). The ruffle will minimize the size of the hand
c. loose bracelets

d. large rings
e. nails medium length, well-cared for; medium shades of polish

AVOID:

a. long sleeves that are too short
b. delicate jewelry
c. bare hands (no polish or jewelry)
d. short fingernails

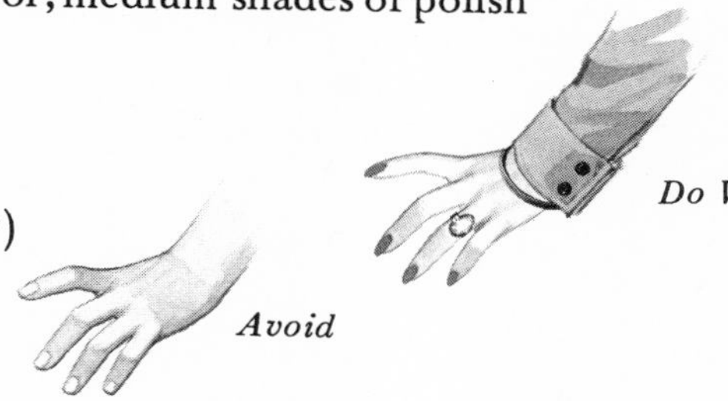

Do Wear

Avoid

HIPS

Too Wide and Too Large

DO WEAR:

a. overblouses, tops worn "out"
b. top with bottom (if your upper half is not as large as the bottom)
c. suits with capes or jackets extending down just past largest point of hips (such as box jackets to balance hips)
d. medium- to lightweight fabrics which fall gracefully over hips, but do not cling
e. dull-finish fabrics
f. vertical lines in fabric and garment designs on lower garments
g. box jackets, vests, boleros, or layered upper garments to balance
h. styles that emphasize small waist (but if you are short, no belts of different colors)
i. slightly flared skirts
j. dark lower garments (light top if medium to tall)
k. A-line dresses

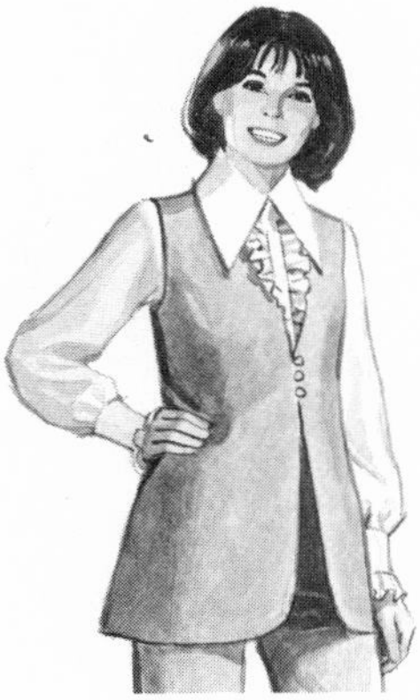

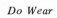

Do Wear

AVOID:

a. Empire-style tops or dresses
b. waistlines that are too nipped in
c. belts that are too wide or contrasting in color
d. below-waistline trimming
e. very short skirts or shorts
f. full, gathered, or pleated skirts
g. very straight or clingy skirts or slacks
h. patch pockets near hip line
i. white or very light colors on lower garments
j. shiny or flimsy skirt or slacks fabrics
k. long fitted jackets that go over the hips
l. bold colors or large-print fabrics on lower half of body

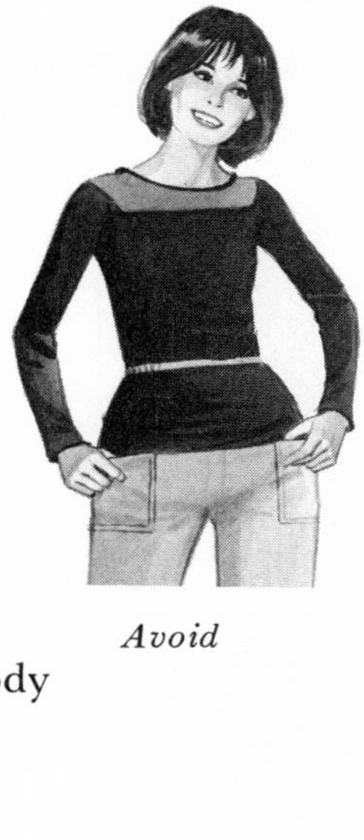

Avoid

Too Narrow and Too Bony

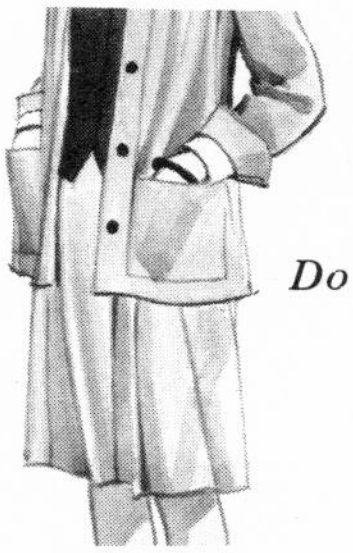

Do Wear

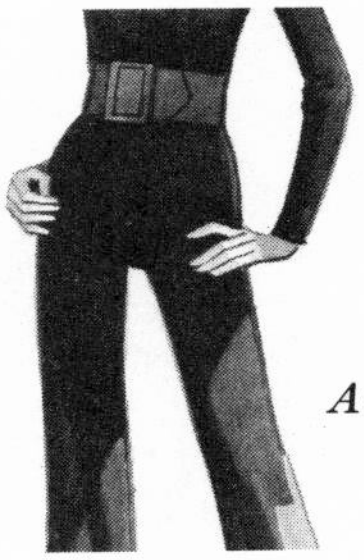

Avoid

DO WEAR:

a. extra half-slip or pettipants with skirts or pants (to give the illusion of more flesh underneath the clothing)
b. jackets or sweaters which extend past waist to middle of hips
c. shirtwaist dresses
d. pleated or gathered skirts with draping or shirring
e. full-cut slack styles
f. medium- to heavyweight fabrics
g. light or bright colors with plaids and other patterns, horizontal designs on lower garments
h. oversized and decorated pockets on pants and skirts

AVOID:

a. skimpy, clingy skirts and pants made out of materials such as jersey
b. straight-line or pencil-slim skirts and slacks
c. vertical design in garment or fabric design
d. dark colors on lower half of body, when possible

KNEES

Too Bony

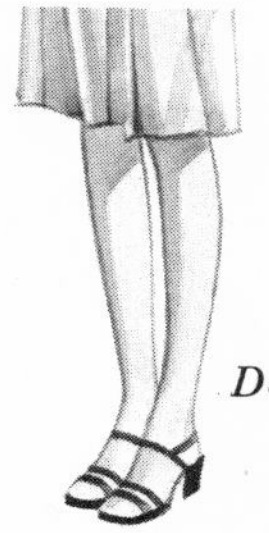

Do Wear

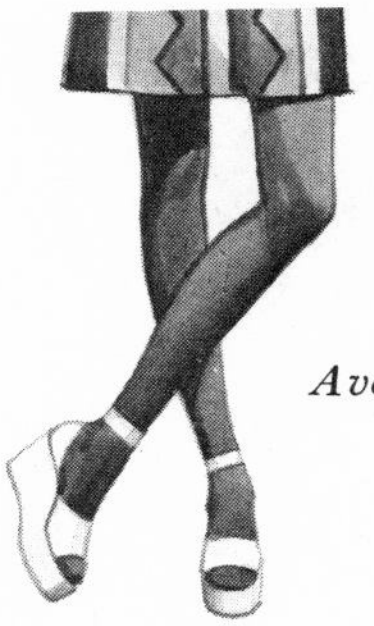

Avoid

DO WEAR:

a. dresses and skirts just below the knee
b. slacks, knickers, culottes, pedal pushers, whenever possible
c. simple, graceful shoes—open-toe and back, sandals, low cut
d. stockings and tights (they have a tendency to soften the bony knee)

AVOID:

a. dresses and skirts above or just above your knee caps
b. short shorts, regular shorts
c. awkward, cumbersome shoes

Knock-Knees

DO WEAR:

a. dresses and skirts at least ½ inch below the knees
b. slacks when and if possible
c. shorts, pedal pushers, gauchos, culottes, at least 2 inches below the knee
d. medium-tone stockings
e. shoe styles that are not exaggerated or extreme or clunky

AVOID:

a. dresses and skirts above or right at the knee
b. skinny-type slacks
c. when possible, stockings or tights in too light or too dark a tone

LEGS

Too Heavy

DO WEAR:

a. medium-length skirts (below the calf) which have medium-full bottom (A-line, slight gather, slight pleat); this gives the illusion of a thinner leg
b. floor-length skirts and dresses
c. Bermuda-style, rather than short shorts
d. vertically designed garments and fabrics for lower part of body
e. medium-to-dark shades of brown- and gray-tone stockings
f. shoe, stockings, and lower garment color should blend for best effect
g. higher-heeled shoes
h. shoe with open toe or open heel

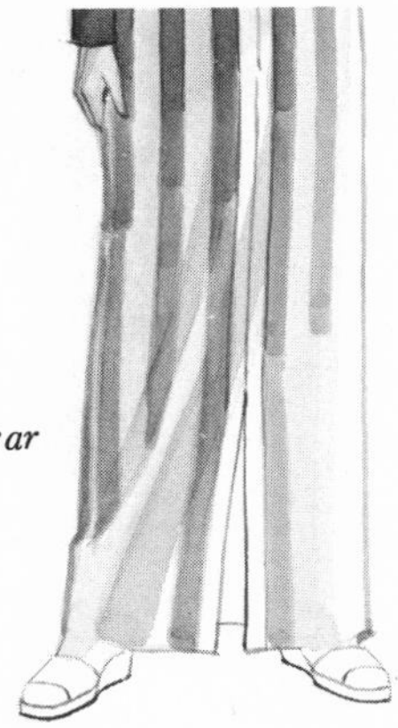

Do Wear

AVOID:

a. skirts that stop above or at the knee
b. slacks that fit too tightly
c. short shorts
d. light-colored, patterned, or novelty color stockings—this only emphasizes your problem
e. strap-style shoes that are too delicate

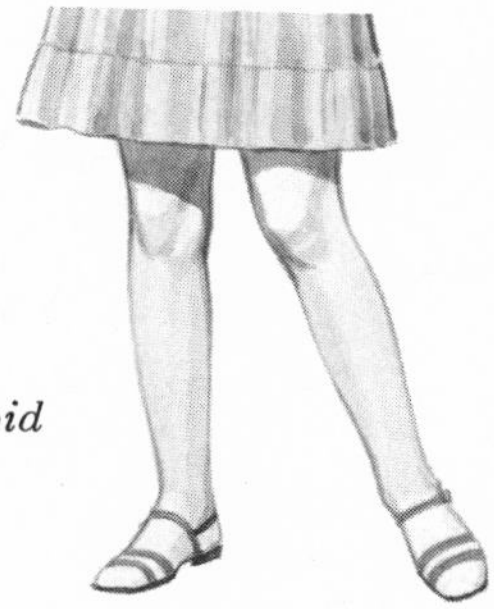

Avoid

Too Thin

DO WEAR:

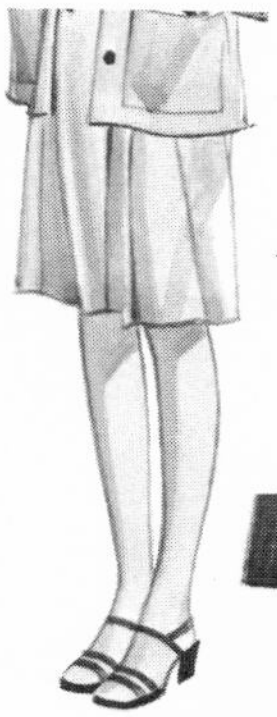
Do Wear

a. slacks of medium- to heavyweight fabrics
b. horizontal garment and fabric designs in skirts and slacks
c. dresses and skirts that fall gracefully near the legs
d. slacks with legs not too tight
e. light color slacks and skirts
f. Bermuda-style, rather than short shorts
g. hem lengths around the knee, or an inch or two below
h. pedal pushers, knickers, culottes, etc., on the form-fitting rather than full side
i. light shades of stockings, tights
j. simple, delicate shoes—low cut, slingback, open toe

AVOID:

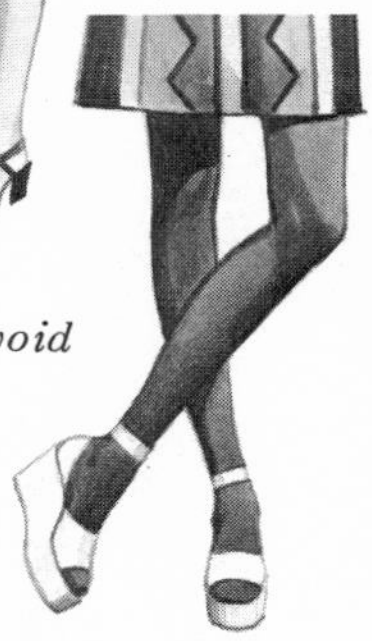
Avoid

a. street-length dresses that are overly full at the bottom
b. very short shorts, dresses, and skirts
c. A-line skirts and dresses
d. solid, dark-color fabrics in any type of garment
e. overly tight or clingy slacks and skirts
f. darker-colored stockings
g. oversized shoes that make your legs look even smaller

Bowed

DO WEAR:

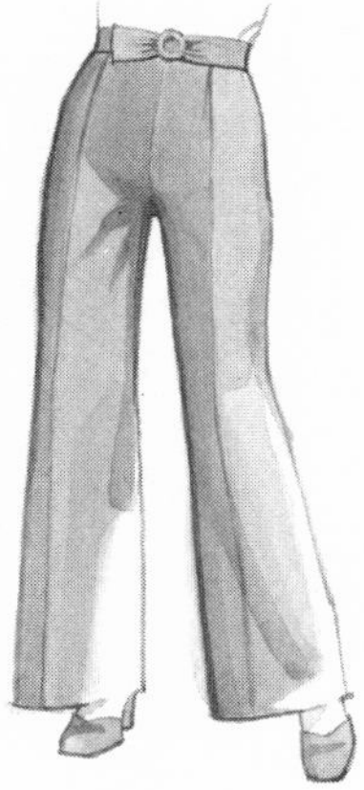
Do Wear

a. dresses and skirts just past the largest point of your bow, whenever possible
b. slacks (if you have the figure for them)
c. long dresses whenever possible
d. low-cut shoes

AVOID:

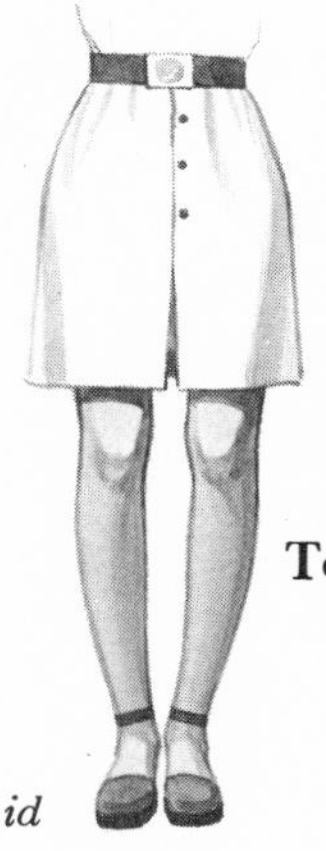
Avoid

a. dress length above or just below the knees (just a bit longer)
b. slacks with tight or clingy legs
c. shorts, etc., above the largest point of your bow
d. ankle-strap shoes
e. shoes that come up to the ankle area

Too Short

DO WEAR:

a. skirts, slacks, dresses with vertical design emphasis
b. skirts just above the knee or just touching it

c. high-top slacks (waistbands extending above your natural waist), or a wide belt if your entire body is not short
d. pants or skirts well-tailored around hips, becoming slightly fuller toward hem
e. short shorts (the shorter, the better)
f. higher heels on shoes (make sure slacks or long skirt cover most of shoe)

AVOID:

a. wide belts if your total appearance is short
b. ruffles, flounces, or any large detail on skirts or slacks
c. hip huggers
d. slacks with cuffs—the straighter the line of the slacks, the longer your legs will appear
e. slacks that drag the floor (you will look as if you are trying to grow into them)
f. large prints
g. horizontal designs in fabric and garment design

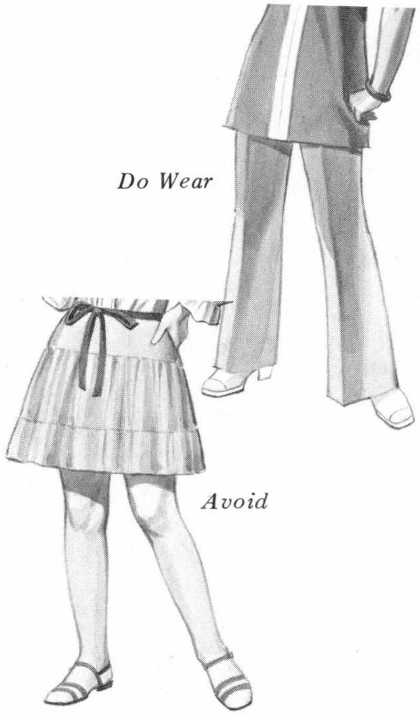

Do Wear

Avoid

Too Long

DO WEAR:

a. skirts just below the knee
b. wide belts (unless you are short-waisted)
c. jackets, sweaters, and other garments that extend below the waist
d. hip huggers
e. slacks that are long enough for you
f. slacks with cuffs
g. contrasting colors in upper and lower garments
h. horizontal garment and fabric design (unless you have an overall heaviness problem)
i. shorts with cuffs
j. knickers, pedal pushers, culottes, gauchos, if at least 2 inches below the knee

AVOID:

a. waistbands that look to be above normal waistline
b. pants that are just a bit too short for you
c. vertical fabric and garment design
d. extremely high heels

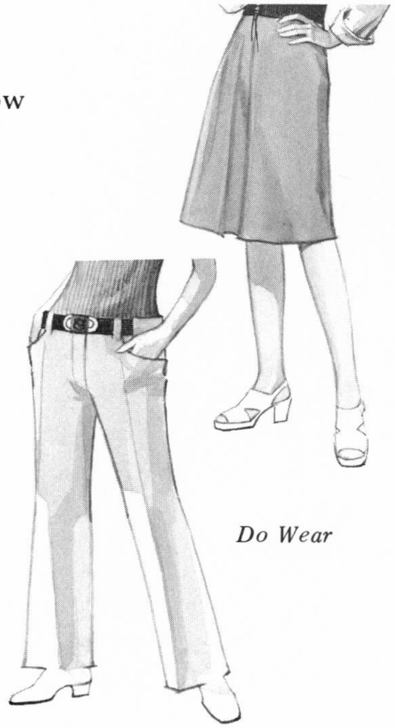

Do Wear

Heavy Thighs

(see "Hips, Too Wide and Too Large" and "Thighs: Upper Thighs, Bulges, Rolls")

NECK

Bony, Too Long, Too Thin

DO WEAR:

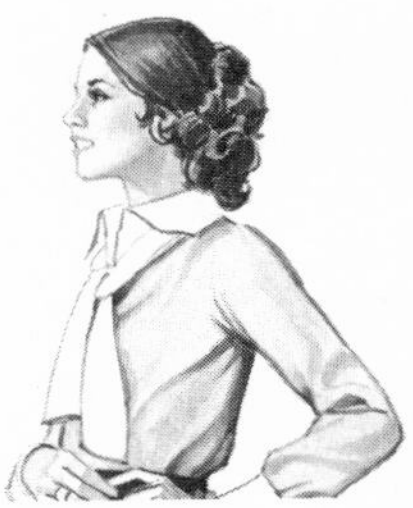

Do Wear

a. hair close to shoulder length (or longer if you wish)
b. high necklines to break the length of neck
c. fussy high necklines, such as big bows, ornate collars, ruffles
d. high scoop necklines with delicate jewelry
e. layered necklines (slipover garment worn over shirtwaist blouse; V-neck garments over turtleneck)
f. scarves or jewelry if you have a V- or deep-cut garment (see Accessories, Chapter Eight)

AVOID:

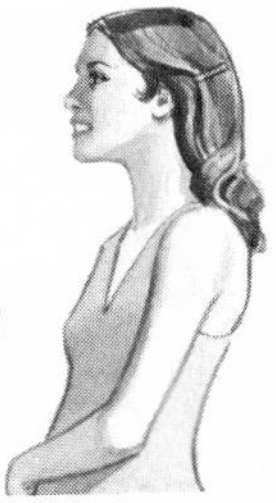

Avoid

a. upsweep or short hair styles—longer hair will give you a much softer look. If you do wear your hair in an upsweep, be sure to break your neckline by wearing very high collars, turtlenecks, or high ruffles
b. deep V-neckline (unless length of neck is broken with use of jewelry, scarf, or maybe a flower), or low scoop garments
c. garments that leave the whole length of the neck and upper chest exposed

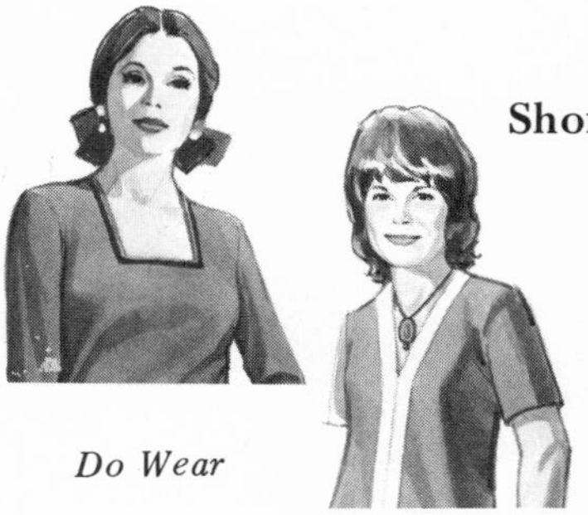

Do Wear

Short or Plump

DO WEAR:

a. hair up or away from your neck
b. simple necklines—the simpler, the better
c. V-neck garments

d. low necklines
e. soft fabrics in high neckline styles (if you must wear them at all)

AVOID:

a. hairstyles that will cover up all of neck
b. anything fussy at the neck; this covers it up and gives the impression that you have no neck
c. high-neck styles (unless very simple and soft)
d. scarves around neck
e. jewelry on the neck; wear drop jewelry away from neck
f. bulky turtlenecks

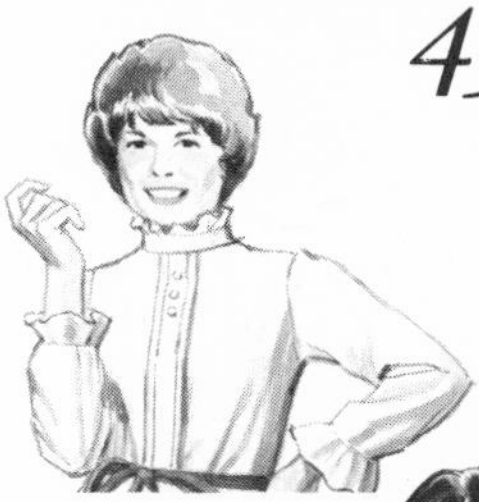

Avoid

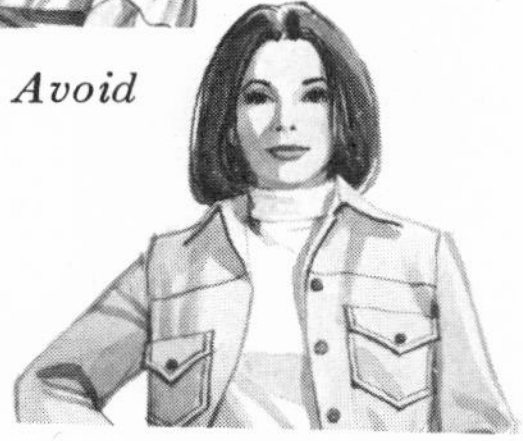

RIB CAGE

Too Small

DO WEAR:

a. upper garments of medium- to heavyweight fabrics that will drape or fall nicely from the bust down to the waist
b. anything horizontal across the rib cage
c. horizontal garment and fabric designs in blouses, sweaters, and other such garments
d. the layered look

AVOID:

a. garments that fit tightly between bust and waistline
b. fabrics that are too clingy

Do Wear

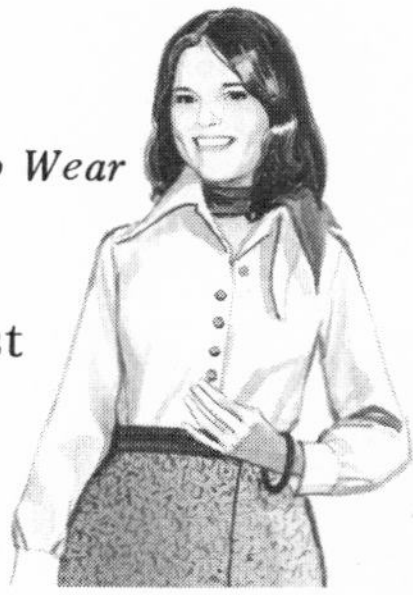

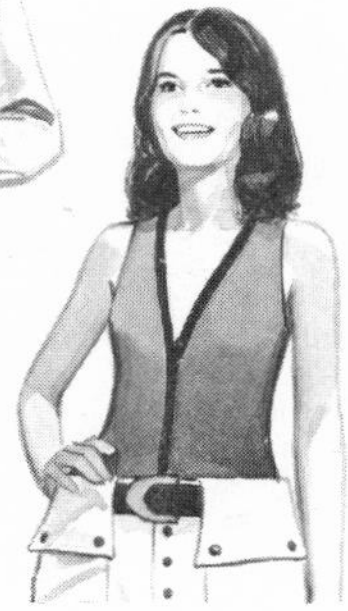

Avoid

Too Large

DO WEAR:

a. tailored-type blouses; the more fabric you "take away," the slimmer you appear. Take extra darts if necessary
b. garments with vertical seams set in from each side
c. vertical fabric designs
d. two-piece dresses with easy overblouse and a slightly gathered skirt for best overall effect

AVOID:

a. full blouses or sweaters
b. upper garments that are extremely tight or clingy
c. horizontal garment and fabric design in upper garments
d. fabrics that are overly bulky

Do Wear

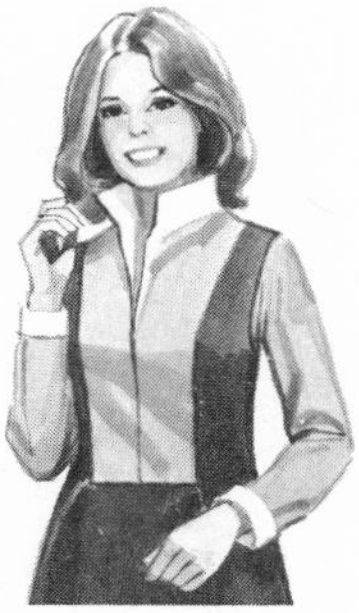

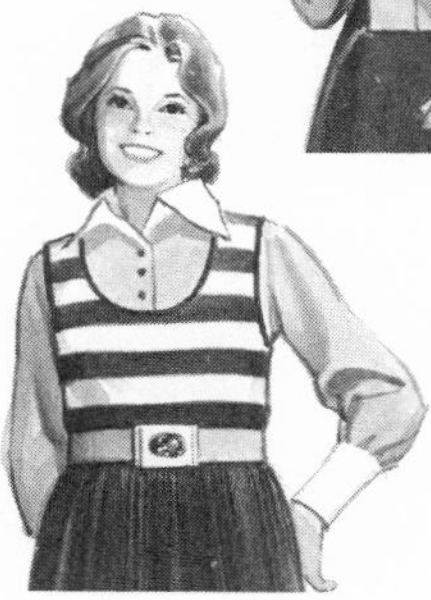

Avoid

SHOULDERS

Too Wide

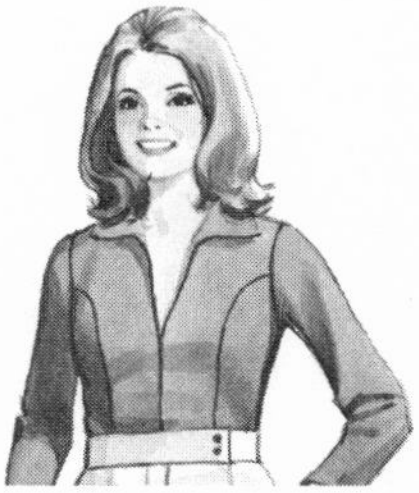

Do Wear

DO WEAR:

a. tailored, smooth garments on shoulders
b. shoulder seams slightly inside actual edge of shoulder line
c. closely fitted upper garments with vertical seams set in from each side
d. vests and boleros with large armholes coming in toward center of body
e. raglan sleeves (and other styles that "break" the shoulder line)
f. fabrics with vertical designs as much as possible
g. dark colors on upper half of body

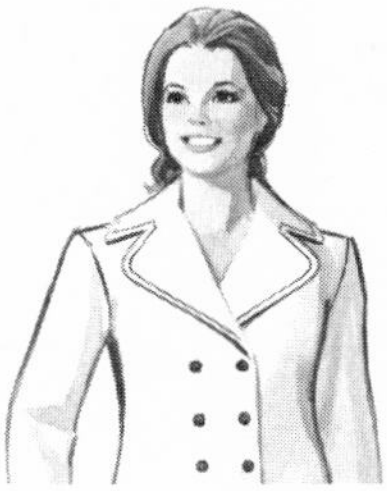

Avoid

AVOID:

a. shoulder pads at all times
b. any gathering at shoulders, such as puffy or other fussy sleeves
c. sweaters and tops that are too tight and clingy
d. double-breasted styles
e. garments that are a little too large for you
f. horizontal lines in garment design and fabric design

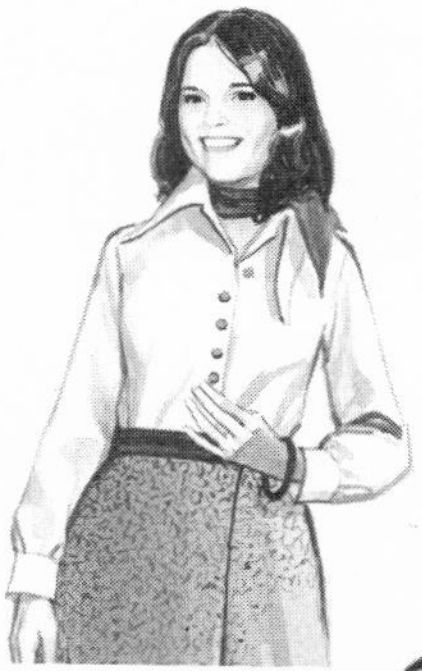

Do Wear

Too Narrow

DO WEAR:

a. soft shoulder pads, scarves, wide collars at shoulder line
b. extended shoulder line, crosswise yokes
c. shoulder seams just on the other side of the shoulder
d. puffy and fussy sleeves near the shoulder
e. short sleeves, cap sleeves, short puff sleeves, sleeves that extend slightly out onto the shoulder
f. horizontal lines in fabric and garment design

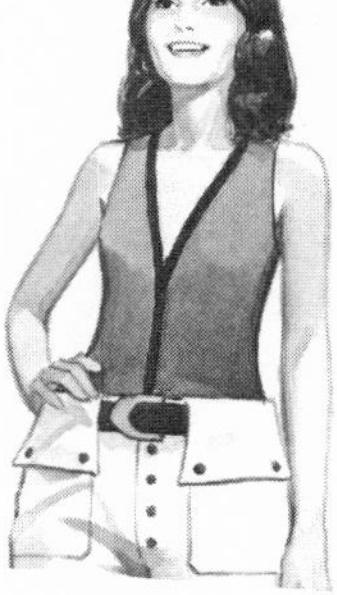

Avoid

AVOID:

a. tight, clingy garments on upper half of body
b. vests, boleros, or any other garment that would tend to focus the attention in toward the center of the body
c. kimono and raglan sleeves
d. vertical garment and fabric design

Sloping or Round

Round shoulders that are strictly a posture defect can be corrected with some consistent effort.

DO WEAR:

a. high scoops and V-necks
b. soft shoulder pads when possible
c. extended shoulder line, crosswise yokes
d. puffy and fussy sleeves near the shoulder
e. jackets and the layered look

AVOID:

a. large scoop necks that extend outward to the shoulder
b. halter-style tops
c. sleeveless tops
d. vests, boleros, or any other garment that would tend to focus the attention in toward the center of the body
e. kimono and raglan sleeves
f. vertical garment and fabric design

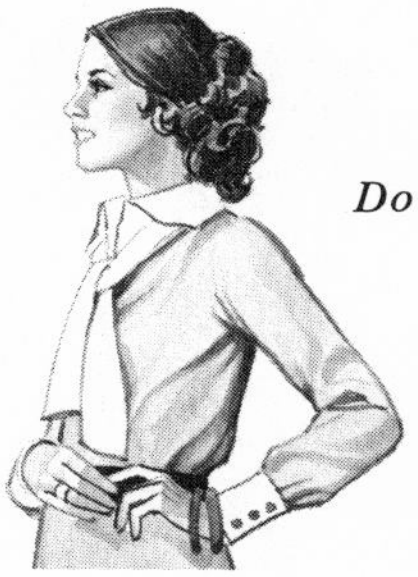

Do Wear

Shoulder Blades Protruding

DO WEAR:

a. clothing loosely fitted across the shoulder blades
b. jackets, vests, boleros, the layered look

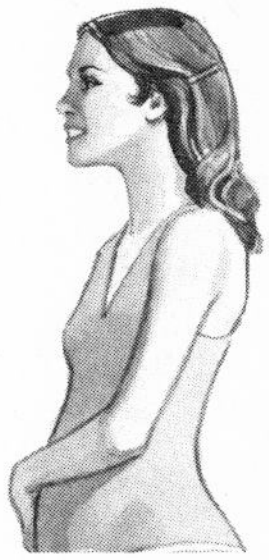

Avoid

AVOID:

a. thin, tightly fitted fabrics across shoulder blades
b. deep-cut styles in the back, unless you have long hair to soften the look

STOMACH

Too Full

DO WEAR:

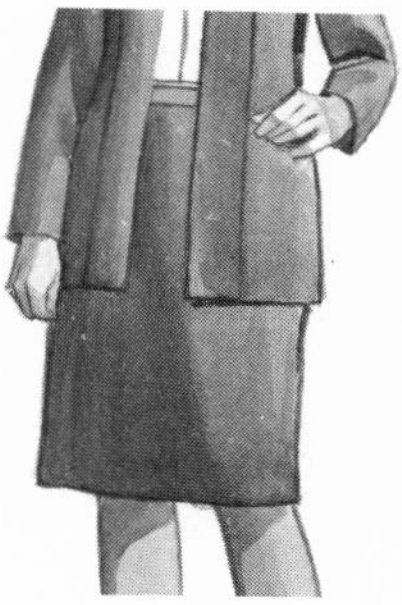

Do Wear

a. the proper control undergarment (see Chapter Seven)
b. overblouses, tunic-style tops
c. belts slightly on the narrow and loose side (do not pull in too tightly as your stomach will appear fuller)
d. garments that fit loosely across the stomach; if they are too tight, the stomach tends to be exaggerated
e. A-line, princess styles, darker color skirts and pants
f. slightly flared skirts
g. darts in the front of garments, over the stomach (rather than tucks or gathers), to make a smooth line at the waist
h. flat front zippers, or wear zipper in back if possible

AVOID:

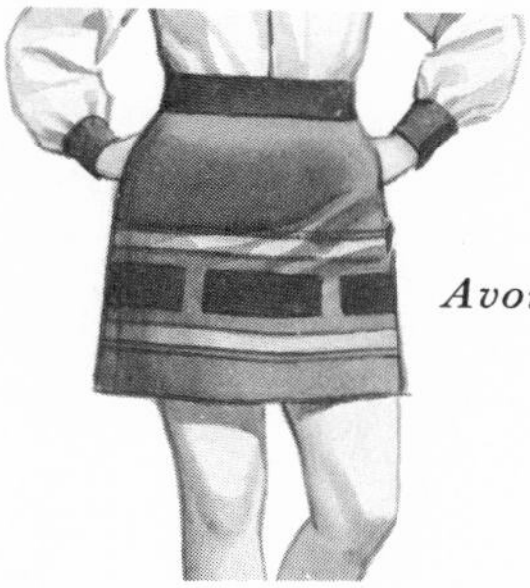

Avoid

a. Empire styles
b. tight waistband styles of dress or top
c. wide or tight belts
d. garments that are too loose and flowing across the stomach, such as gathered skirts; they will add to the largeness of it
e. garments that fit too tightly under the stomach
f. gored skirts
g. zippered fronts, especially ones thick with fabric
h. any tight slacks; hip huggers
i. pants styles with trim or decoration (including belt loops, etc.) at the waist or over the stomach

THIGHS: UPPER THIGHS, BULGES, ROLLS

(see also Hips, Too Wide and Too Large)

DO WEAR:

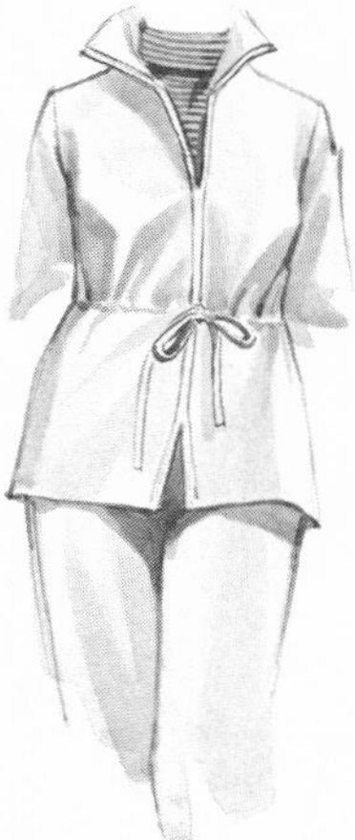

Do Wear

a. jackets that come to the top of the largest area of the bulge
b. skirts and dresses that fall near the knee
c. slightly flared skirts, A-line
d. very slight pleat or draping effect
e. full-cut leg styles of slacks

f. pedal pushers, knickers, culottes, gauchos, with a slight fullness
g. dark lower garments
h. vertical lines in fabric and garment designs on lower garments
i. medium to lightweight fabrics that fall gracefully over thighs, but do not cling

AVOID:

a. very short skirts, short shorts
b. very straight or clingy skirts or slacks
c. tight-fitting pants (which tend to exaggerate rolls or bulges)
d. pockets or decoration around the thigh area
e. light colors on lower garments

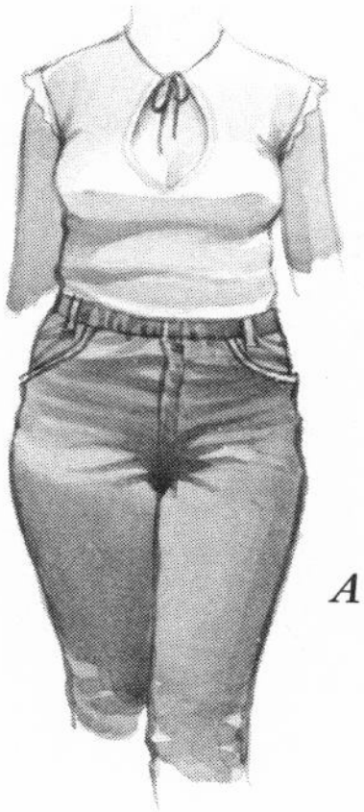

Avoid

Do Wear

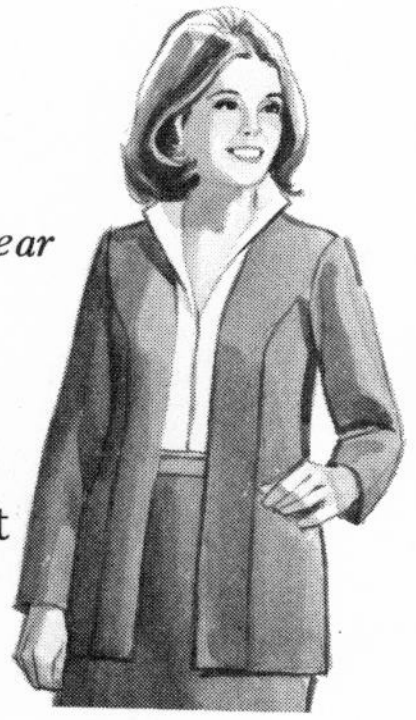

WAIST

The Average or Heavy Girl With Too Large a Waist

DO WEAR:

a. soft overblouse or sweater
b. jackets that extend to hips
c. soft slim belt that ties one time
d. a waist cincher for that special dress or outfit (see Chapter Seven)
e. fabrics that fall gracefully from waist—not too tight or baggy
f. solid medium-to-dark colors

AVOID:

a. wide belts or waistbands
b. high waistband or tight, wide midriff-band dress styles
c. gathered or pleated skirts
d. large, bright prints
e. pockets, belt loops, and other decorative trim at the waist

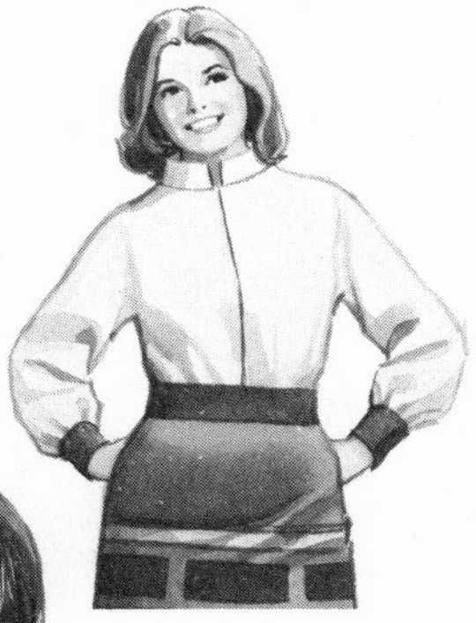

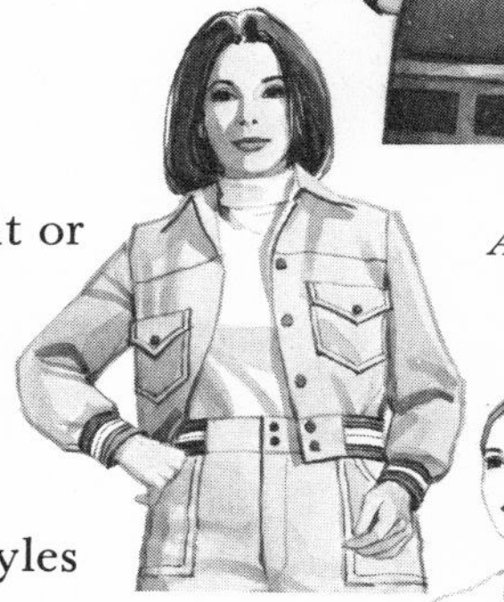

Avoid

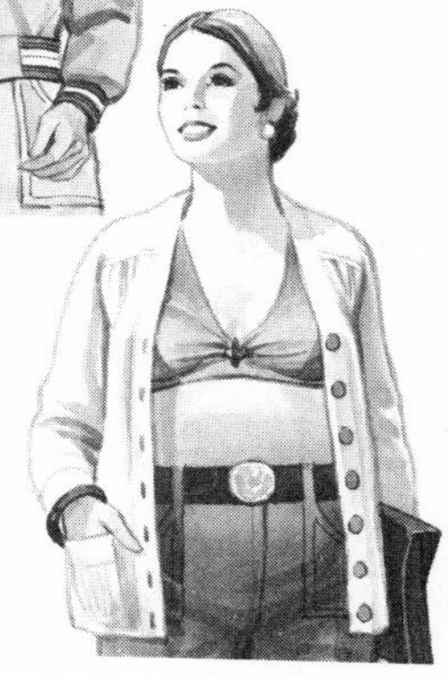

The Thin Girl With Too Large a Waist

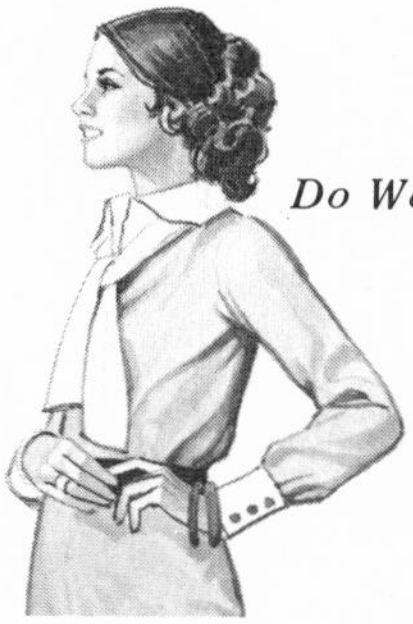

Do Wear

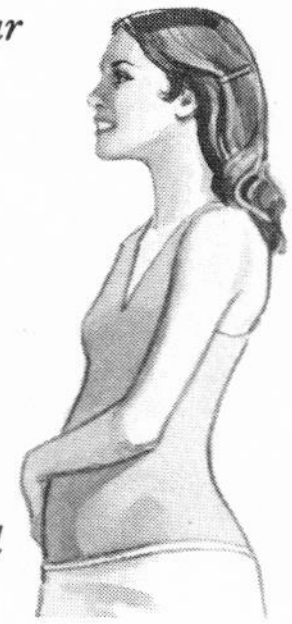

Avoid

DO WEAR:

a. clothing above waist slightly on the loose side (which makes the waist appear smaller)
b. belts to "bring in" the waist (narrow ones if you are short)
c. skirts or dresses that are full just below the waist

AVOID:

a. skin-tight clothing just below and above the waist
b. wide belts unless you are over 5′8″

WRISTS

Too Bony, Too Thin

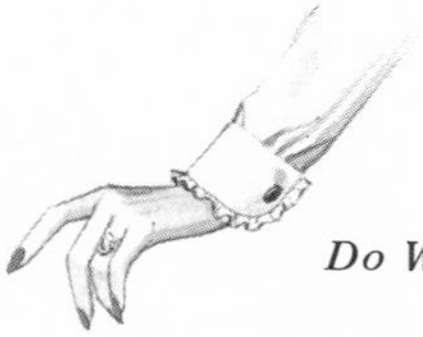

Do Wear

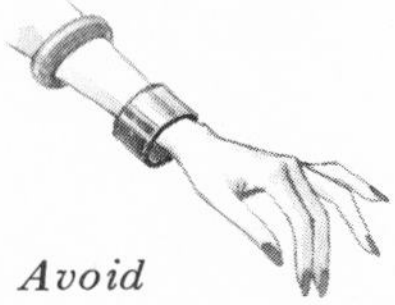

Avoid

DO WEAR:

a. long sleeves a little past the wrist bone
b. ruffles or lace on sleeve around wrist
c. delicate jewelry on wrist

AVOID:

a. puffy or very full sleeves that stop between your elbow and wrist
b. oversized jewelry for your arm

Too Thick

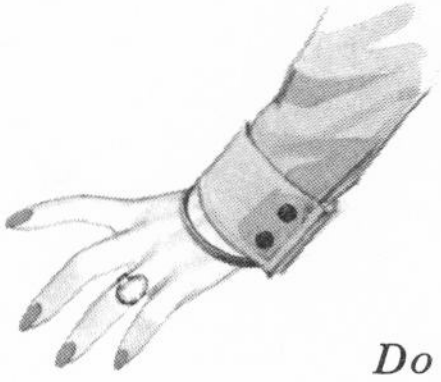

Do Wear

DO WEAR:

a. long sleeves almost touching the hand
b. wide or bulky bracelets
c. several small or thin bracelets at once
d. wide watchbands

AVOID:

a. 3/4-length sleeves
b. skimpy, clingy, too-short long sleeves
c. delicate jewelry unless wearing several pieces together

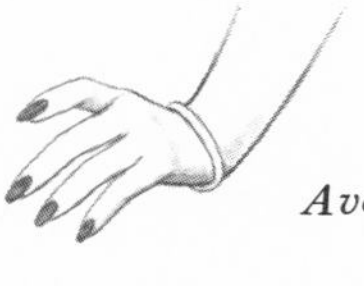

Avoid

Chapter Four

BALANCING COMBINATION PROBLEMS

A combination problem generally means that your upper torso and lower torso are "out of balance." Balancing combination problems is an old, old trick and is used by actresses and TV personalities (and yes, even by some models) ALL THE TIME. Many of them are so skillful at camouflaging their defects that you don't know what their problems are. They have succeeded in giving the illusion of a more perfect figure. This is not really difficult to do and is an art well worth mastering.

First turn back to Chapter Two and study carefully your Proportion Chart. Once you know your specific problem (and it's most likely you will have only one of the combination problems), you can then start making good use of your full-length mirror—checking front, back, and side views. There are so many ways that you can balance your figure with clothing by accentuating the positive and subtly eliminating the "negative."

For example, if your Proportion Chart shows you to be too large in one area for the proportion of other parts of your body, here's what to do: wear styles and fabrics that do not add to the width of that area. Also wear garments that lay close to the *largest points* of that particular area. Then, balance the other parts of the body with clothing that fits a little looser. Or, if possible, wear the layered look on the smaller area.

Let's look at six common problems of proportion. Find YOUR problem and give the illusion of a better figure by following the do's and don'ts.

LONG-WAISTED (Shorter legs with longer body)

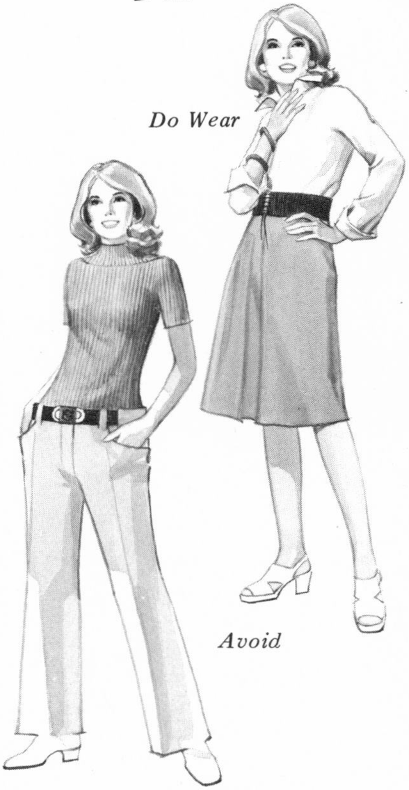

Do Wear

Avoid

DO WEAR:

a. waistbands slightly higher than your waist. No one but you can tell exactly where your real waist is located unless you have on a bikini. When you buy pants, skirts, and dresses, pick out garments that have just the right height waistband for you and get used to the feeling of the waistband being higher than normal
b. high-waisted garments with one or more belts, which help break the expanse between the bustline and the hips
c. an undefined waistline with soft sweaters, long knitted evening gown
d. wide belts, sashes, and wide, horizontally designed fabric belts (if you are slim) that are worn slightly above the waist
e. long dresses and skirts when possible (with the higher-than-normal waistband mentioned above). This gives the illusion of longer legs and a more flowing line between waistband and feet
f. skirts and dresses (for street wear) near the knee, rather than too short—this helps make the space between waist and knee appear to be longer than it is

AVOID:

a. clinging blouses and sweaters
b. small, narrow belts at *regular* waistline
c. loose low waistlines of any kind (including the "flapper look")
d. hip huggers (pants made with the waistband at least 2 inches below your waistline). They make your legs look shorter, which in turn makes your waist look even longer
e. above-the-knee skirts or pants

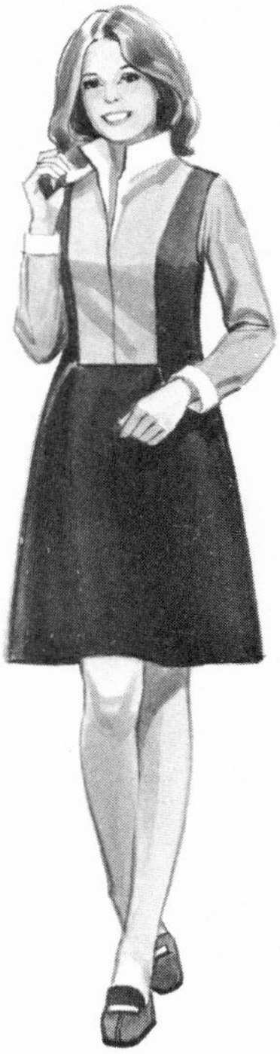

SHORT-WAISTED (Long legs with short midriff)

DO WEAR:

a. hats with height or an upward sweep
b. stand-up collar
c. a long continuous scarf from neck past waistline
d. overblouses, two-piece overlayer outfits
e. unbelted princess lines, Empire silhouettes

Do Wear

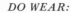

f. narrow belts below normal waistline
g. garments with waistband slightly below your normal waist; hip huggers
h. vertical or diagonal fabrics and designs, unbroken from shoulder to hem when possible

AVOID:

a. waistlines that are high or built-up
b. wide belts
c. skirts that are box-pleated or gathered, if you are short and short-waisted. This destroys the illusion you are trying to create of a longer torso
d. garments that are too thick and layered through the middle—this accentuates even more the small expanse between bust and hips

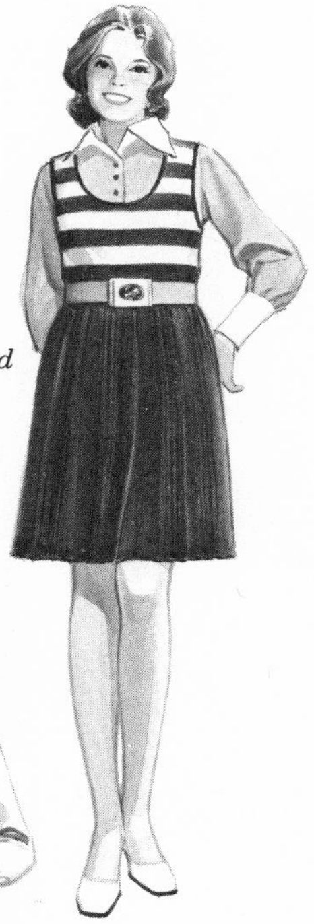

Avoid

BROAD HIPS—NARROW SHOULDERS

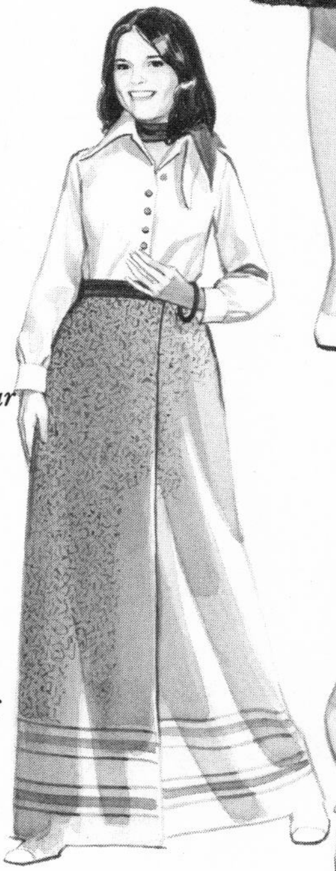

Do Wear

DO WEAR:

a. collars extended past the shoulder line
b. soft shoulder pads when possible
c. shawls
d. top sleeve seam with gathers
e. A-line skirts
f. darker colors on lower part of body, lighter on top
g. vertical designs in fabric and garment design on lower half of body

AVOID:

a. sleeves set farther in than regular shoulder line
b. vests or sleeveless jackets that are wider at waist than at neck
c. vertical fabric or garment design on top half of body
d. gathered and box-pleated skirts
e. horizontal designs on lower half of body
f. fabrics that are bulky on hips
g. hip or patch pockets on pants, skirts, shorts (any garment worn on lower part of body)

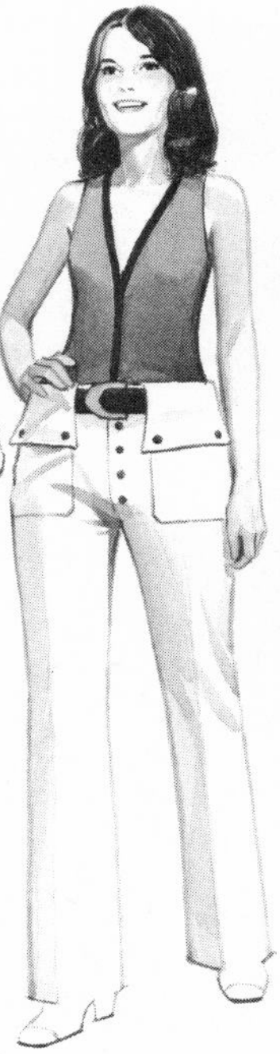

Avoid

NARROW HIPS—BROAD SHOULDERS

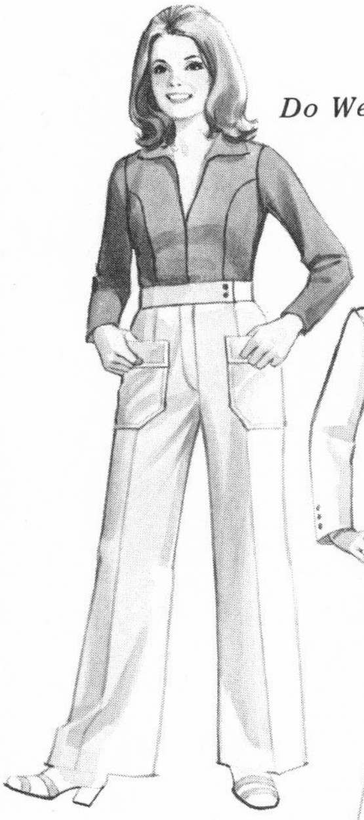

Do Wear

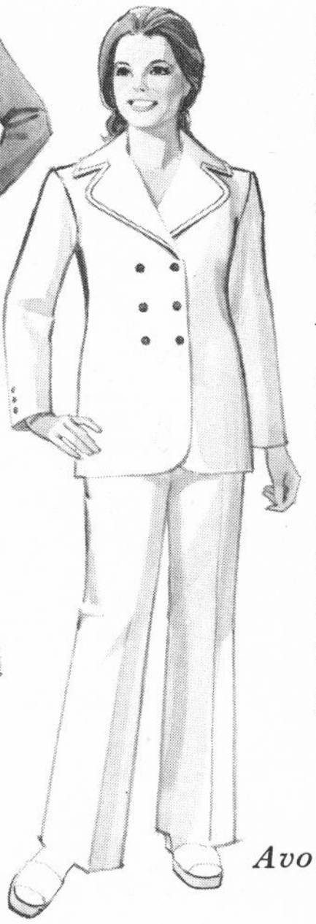

Avoid

DO WEAR:

a. loose, full hair or brimmed hat
b. V-neck lines
c. front-button-down tops
d. single-breasted jackets
e. gathered or pleated skirts and dresses
f. darker colors on top part of body, lighter on lower part
g. vertical and diagonal fabric designs from shoulders to waist
h. horizontal fabric designs around hips
i. pockets on skirts, pants, dresses at hip line

AVOID:

a. the "pinhead" look (pulled-back, flat-haired look)
b. dress or blouse design with yokes, collars, lapels that give a horizontal feeling
c. jackets or coats with padding in shoulders
d. double-breasted jackets
e. tailored suits
f. pants that are fitted too tightly
g. fabric designs with horizontal lines on lower part of body

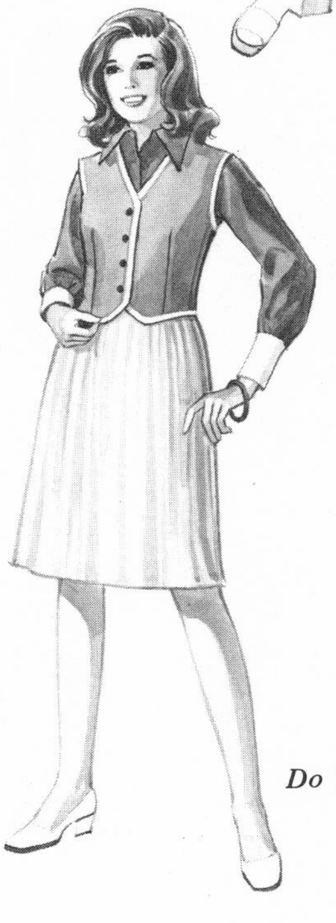

Do Wear

SMALL HIPS—LARGE CHEST

DO WEAR:

a. special brassiere to help give you rounded support instead of the "up" and "out" look (see Chapter Seven)
b. jewelry above or below bust
c. vests or sleeveless boleros (soft fabric)
d. single-breasted jackets
e. softly detailed upper garments
f. dresses and skirts with flared effects that begin at waistline (pleats, gathers)
g. darker-toned blouses and lighter-toned skirts or pants

AVOID:

a. high, round necks
b. frills, big scarves, bows, and other trimming near bust
c. very tight, clinging sweaters, dresses, and blouses
d. white or very light colors from the waist up
e. tight, exaggerated waistlines
f. wide belts

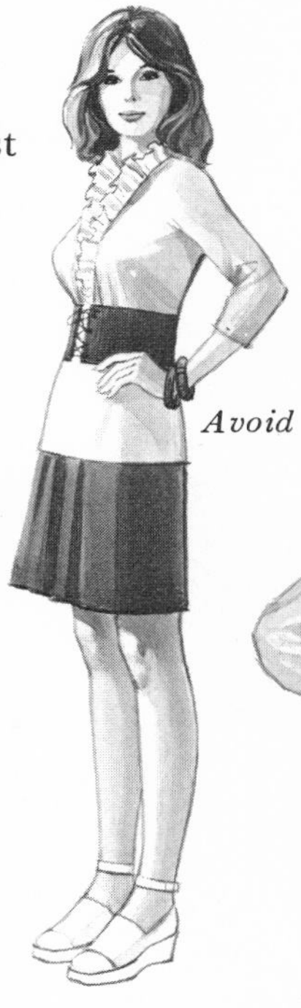

Avoid

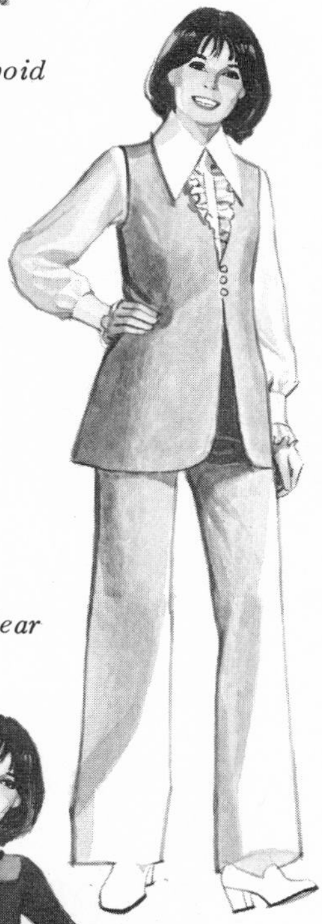

Do Wear

FLAT CHEST–LARGE HIPS

DO WEAR:

a. built-up brassiere
b. scarf or flower at neck to center interest
c. full, feminine blouses
d. tops with shirring, tucks, or pleats
e. vests or boleros
f. the "layered look" on top part of body (blouse with loose sweater or vest on top, left open)
g. light-colored top with dark-colored bottom
h. emphasis on vertical designs in front-center of dress or skirt
i. skirts flaring gently from hips down
j. suits with capes (in winter for an alternative)
k. pantsuits with tunic or medium- to long-length jacket

AVOID:

a. tight-fitting, clingy blouses or sweaters
b. overly tailored blouses
c. gathered or box-pleated skirts and dresses
d. waistbands that are extremely tight or exaggerated
e. very short skirts (these only tend to accentuate the horizontal, chunky lines of the hips)
f. light-colored skirts or slacks
g. horizontal designs around hips

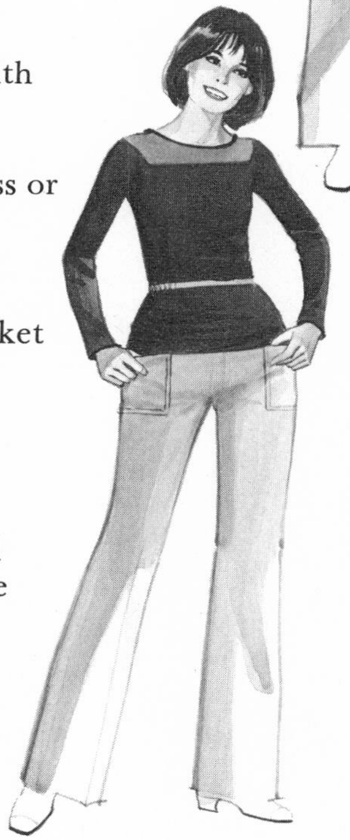

Avoid

Chapter Five

HOW TO LOSE TEN POUNDS IN TEN MINUTES

So you want to look your best for a special occasion and you haven't lost that ten pounds yet? Well, there are ways to give the illusion of weighing less that can give your morale a mighty boost while you are actually getting started on losing that weight. Exactly which techniques you use depend to a certain degree upon your body type.

SHORT AND TOO HEAVY

Proper selection of style, fabric, and accessories can remove many pounds. In dressing to slim down the short and heavy figure, there are two rules to follow: one is to gain as much height as possible (in good taste) and the other is to "remove" the heaviest parts of you by selecting the proper type garments and fabrics. You will shed pounds in minutes. Several famous women fall into the short and heavy category and know very well how to make the most of it . . . SO CAN YOU.

The first picture shows the short, heavy figure as it really is.

The second picture shows the same figure dressed in the wrong type of clothing for that figure; it exaggerates the problems instead of minimizing them.

The third picture shows what proper balance can do. Listed below are many things to avoid so you won't make the mistakes shown in the second picture.

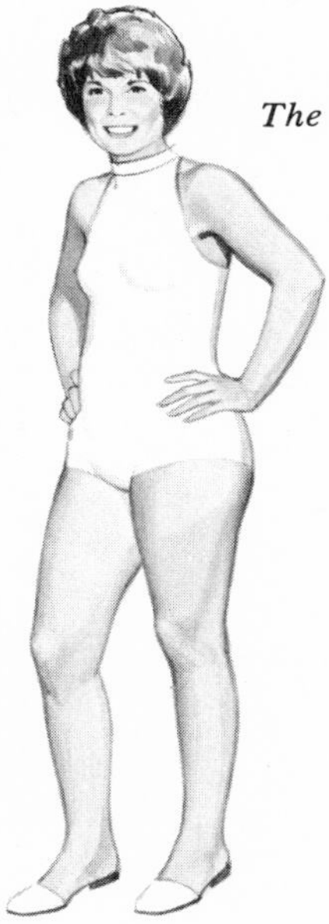

The Short, Heavy Figure

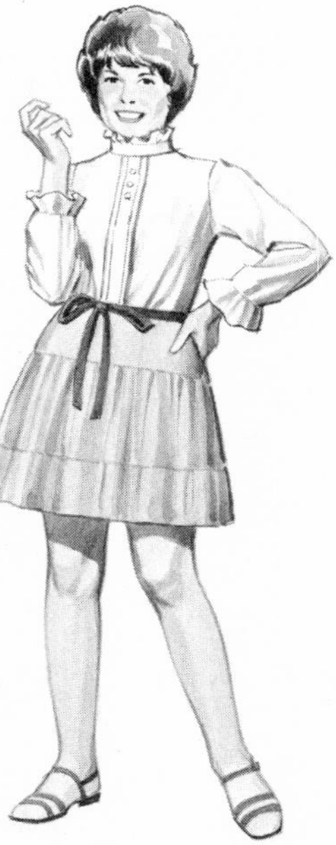

dressed wrong

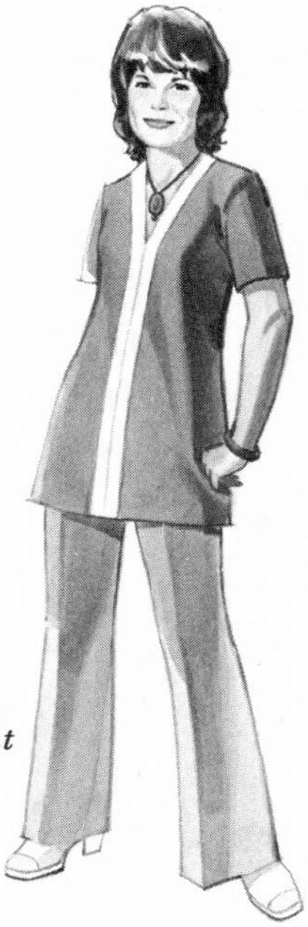

dressed right

AVOID:

a. flat hairstyles
b. turtlenecks (they cut length of neck and make body seem bulkier)
c. overcoats which are double-breasted or with wide lapels (this adds width and decreases height)
d. slim, tight, or straight skirts
e. hems above the knee (the longer and more continuous flow of a skirt or dress, the more height it gives you). But hems should be no longer than 2 inches below the knee, unless they are floor length
f. accessories such as belts and sashes, because they tend to cut into your height

g. "tent" styles
h. rough-textured fabrics such as tweed, heavy wools, or bulky clothing; shiny fabrics
i. horizontal stripes, large patterns, plaids, gathers, pleats, and large patch pockets—all these give width to hips and bust
j. wearing white or light solid colors—this gives the illusion of more width to figure
k. flat shoes

Turning to picture 3, you can see how the following rules apply:

DO WEAR:

a. a hairstyle that gives a little height to your total look. But don't go overboard or you will appear "head heavy"—the balance will be wrong Even if you wear your hair down and just combed out, you can puff the top a bit with subtle teasing
b. correct undergarments (see Chapter Seven)
c. V-necklines (they lengthen the face and neck and give the illusion of greater slenderness)
d. clothes that hug the largest part of your body (but not tightly), such as A-line skirts and dresses; blouses that do not have excess material on the sides; slightly flared skirts
e. smooth lines from shoulder to hem, simple and uncluttered
f. long, narrow lapels on blouses, jackets, and coats (this makes the wearer seem taller)
g. hemlines that fall just below the knee or almost to the floor
h. soft fabrics such as silks, jerseys, soft cottons, soft lightweight synthetics
i. vertically designed fabrics from shoulder to hem; stay with medium- or small-size fabric designs when not able to use a vertical design
j. dark- to medium-color fabrics such as black, brown, navy, dark green, rust
k. medium to dark natural-tone stockings
l. high-heel shoes (but make sure if you're wearing a long skirt, dress, or pants that they are long enough to barely touch the top of shoe and cover most of the heel)

AVERAGE HEIGHT—TOO HEAVY

The average height—too heavy figure has only to be concerned with clothing that "removes" pounds. It's possible to "stretch out" a heavy figure by adding slightly to the top and bottom (hair and shoes). This gives the illusion of being slimmer. Then, with the proper selection of clothing styles and fabrics, you will "remove" inches from your width that will give the illusion of pounds off.

The first picture shows the average height—too heavy figure as it really is.

The second picture shows the same figure with inches added in the wrong place because of the wrong choice of clothing. This woman could instantly remove inches by knowing the right choice of clothing and fabric.

The third picture shows the same figure with proper clothes that give the correct balance. Also, softer fabric helps take away inches.

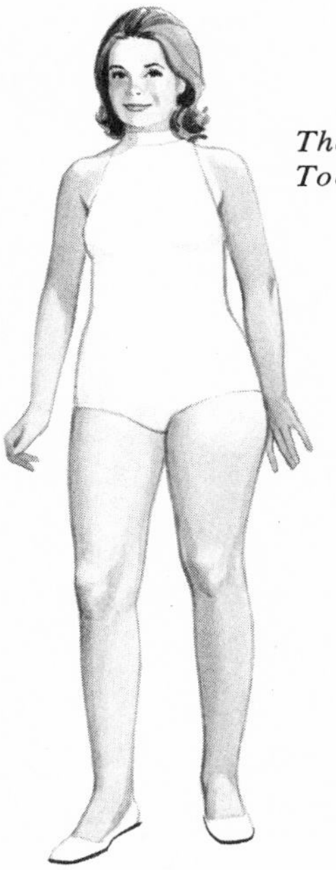

The Average Height, Too Heavy Figure

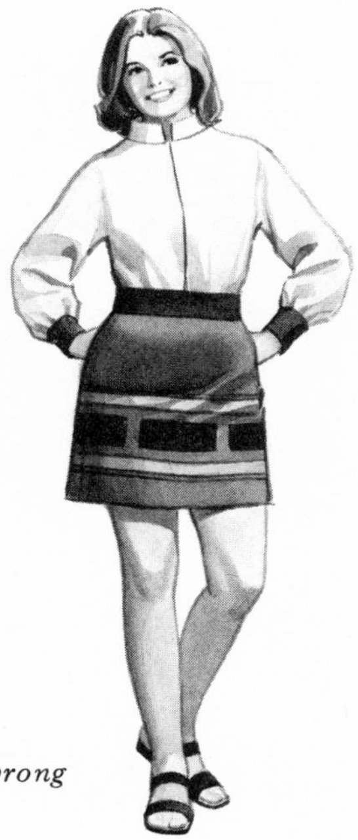

dressed wrong

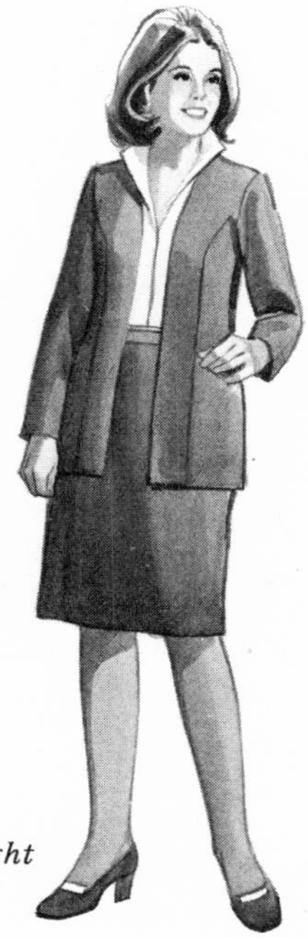

dressed right

AVOID:

a. turtlenecks—they cut length of neck and make the body seem bulkier
b. overcoats that are double-breasted or have wide lapels (this adds width and decreases height)
c. "tent" style tops and dresses
d. if you are exceptionally heavy, avoid belts—an unbroken line will make you appear taller, and therefore slimmer
e. hems above the knee
f. slim, tight, or straight skirts or slacks
g. rough-textured fabrics such as tweed, heavy wools, or bulky clothing; also shiny fabrics
h. white or light solid colors—these give the illusion of more width to the figure
i. horizontal stripes, large or bold patterns, plaids, gathers, pleats, and large patch pockets—all these give width to hips and bust
j. tiny handbags

DO WEAR:

a. a hairstyle with some height will make you appear slimmer; don't make the style top-heavy, though. If your hair is worn hanging down, tease the top ever so slightly at the top-center
b. correct undergarment (see Chapter Seven)
c. V-necks or deep necklines—they lengthen the face and neck and give the illusion of greater slenderness
d. long, narrow lapels on blouses, jackets, and coats—this makes the wearer seem taller
e. smooth lines from shoulder to hem, simple and uncluttered (can be belted)
f. clothes that hug the largest part of your body (but not tightly), such as A-line skirts and dresses; blouses that do not have excess material on the sides; and slightly flared skirts
g. hems should be worn just below the knee
h. medium- to dark-color fabrics (preferably solids such as black, brown, navy, maroon, dark green, etc.), in smooth weaves such as silk, jersey, soft cottons, soft lightweight synthetics; also small- to medium-scale fabric designs
i. high-heel shoes, when possible

TALL AND TOO HEAVY

The tall—too heavy figure can give the illusion of being slimmer and shorter by way of proper choice of garment, fabric, and colors. Movie directors have done this for years when the leading lady was larger or taller than the male lead.

The first picture shows the tall—too heavy figure as it really is.

The second picture shows the same figure dressed in the wrong type of clothing for her. To minimize the problem, look at things to avoid.

The third picture shows how proper balance can improve this type of figure.

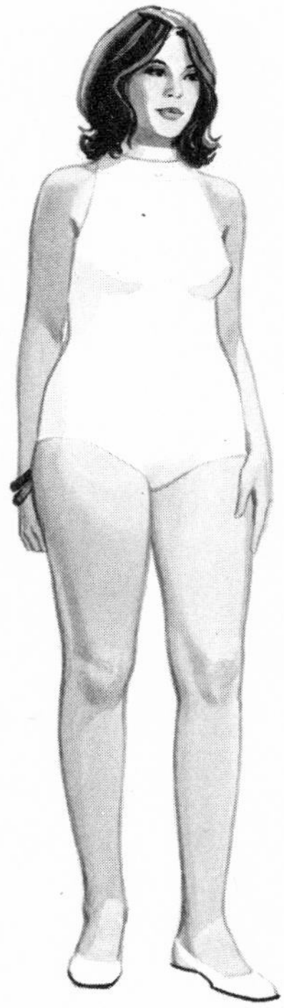

The Tall, Heavy Figure

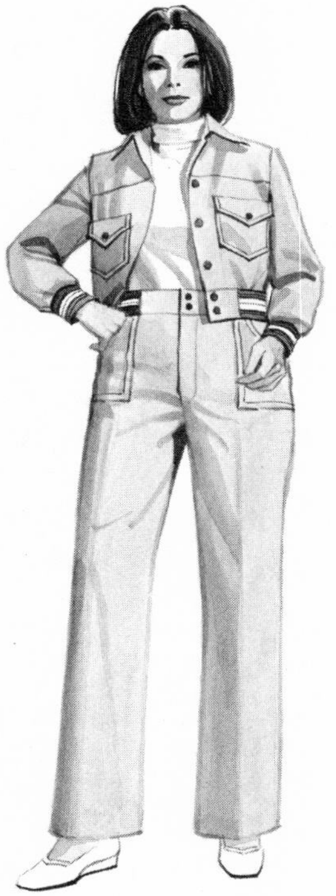

dressed wrong

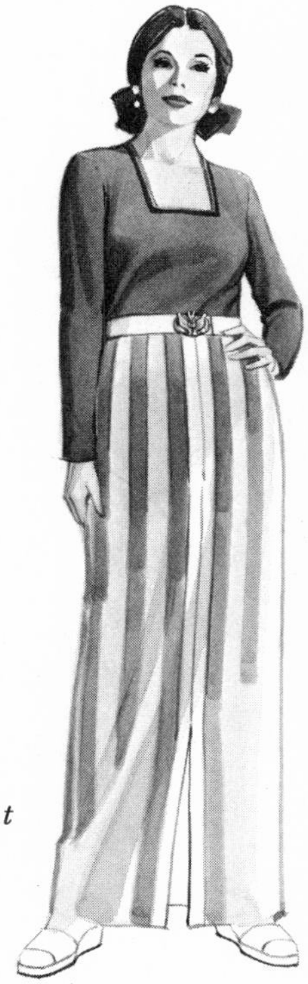

dressed right

AVOID:

a. hairstyles that add more than an inch and a half to your height
b. jewelry that is too small and delicate
c. turtlenecks (they cut length of neck and make body seem bulkier)
d. tent-style tops and dresses

e. overcoats that are double-breasted or have wide lapels (this adds width)
f. slim, tight, or straight skirts
g. hems above the knee (the longer and more continuous flow of a skirt or dress, the more it gives you a slimming effect)
h. clothes too tailored
i. rough-textured fabrics such as tweed, heavy wools, or bulky clothing; also shiny fabrics
j. horizontal stripes, large patterns, plaids, gathers, pleats, and large patch pockets—all these give width to hips and bust
k. white or light solids—this gives the illusion of more width to the figure
l. shoes with platforms or very high heels (over 2 to 2½ inches)

DO WEAR:

a. hairstyle that is soft and does not add more than an inch of height
b. the correct undergarments (see Chapter Seven)
c. jewelry that is large and solid or bulky
d. V- or deep necklines (they lengthen the face and neck and give the illusion of greater slenderness)
e. smooth lines from shoulder to hem, simple and uncluttered (belted if you like)
f. long, narrow lapels on blouses, jackets, and coats (this makes the wearer seem slimmer)
g. clothes that hug the largest part of your body (but not tightly), such as A-line skirts and dresses and blouses that do not have excess material on the sides; and slightly flared skirts
h. narrow belts when possible, to break the height
i. hand or shoulder bag that is medium to large
j. soft fabric weaves such as silks, jerseys, soft cottons, soft lightweight synthetics
k. medium-size fabric designs in deep colors, such as black, navy, brown, dark green
l. medium to dark natural-tone stockings
m. wide-strap sandals and shoes, small heel—instead of delicate sandals

Chapter Six

HOW TO GAIN TEN POUNDS IN TEN MINUTES

If you have an overall thinness problem, you are luckier than you think. You may have a problem for the moment, but it's unlikely that you will have the long-range weight problem of your peers. The too-thin figure is almost a fun problem to solve. You can wear clothing that many would love to be able to wear: bright colors, plaids, bulky and textured knits, the romantic look.

Study the following illustrations and they will help you select the right style, fabric, and accessories for your silhouette. Francey and I would like to add that if you feel you are too thin, enjoy it while you can! Follow these rules and eat all the ice cream and pizza you want, until you have to worry about the *other* side of the coin. We have both been down that road, long ago!

SHORT AND TOO THIN

The first picture shows the short—too thin figure as it really is.

The second picture shows the same figure dressed incorrectly. Adding too much fullness makes the figure appear thinner than it is. Also, the wrong choice of fabric design gives the illusion of appearing shorter.

The third picture shows the result of properly designed ensembles, properly chosen fabrics, hairstyle, and accessories.

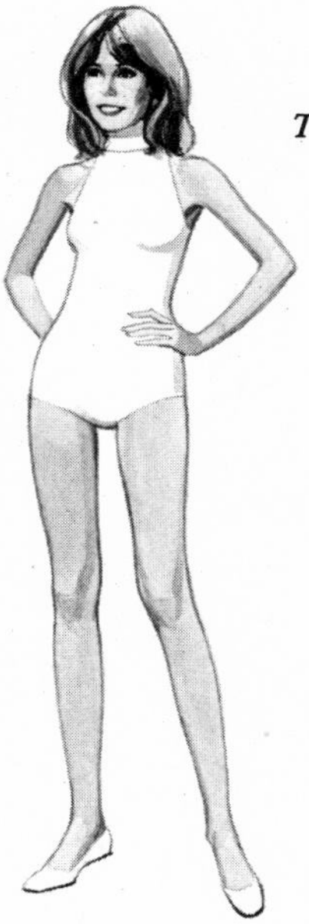

The Short, Thin Figure

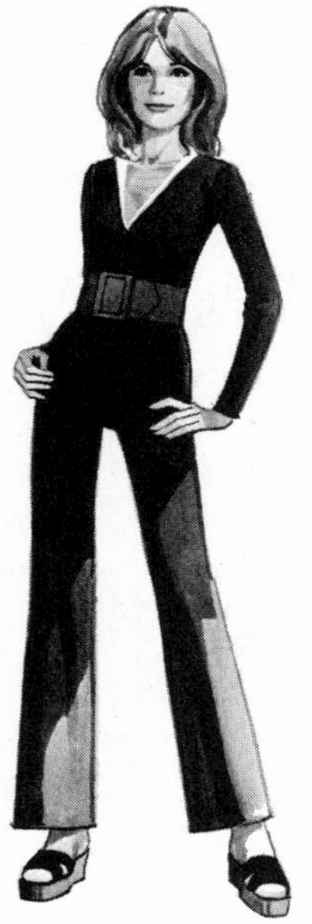

dressed wrong

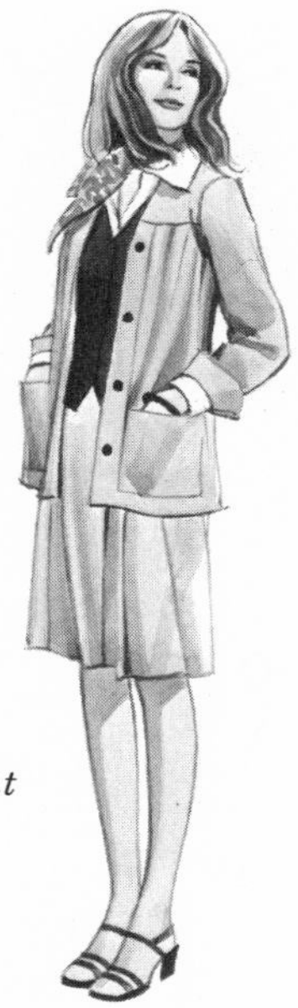

dressed right

AVOID:

a. scoop or wide open necklines
b. any garments too tight, narrow or skimpy
c. sleeveless dresses, unless the shoulder seam is cut in considerably

d. the belted look (belts cut height), especially wide belts
e. boxy or long jackets
f. pencil-slim skirts
g. hems above the knee
h. coats cut full and wide
i. big ruffles or flounces (any heavy or large detail)
j. pants with cuffs
k. big prints and bulky fabrics, two-color ensembles
l. horizontal lines or trimming
m. clinging fabrics, such as jersey
n. dark solid colors

DO WEAR:

a. hairstyles that add an inch or two (do not overdo this as you will look top-heavy and awkward)
b. high necks
c. small scarf to soften thin look around neck
d. simple fullness around bust and hips
e. one-color ensembles (no belts unless it's the same fabric as the outfit); light and bright solid colors to give the illusion of being heavier
f. over-blouses such as sweaters, vests, boleros
g. pants and skirts and tops with pockets; it "adds weight"
h. fitted coats and suit jackets
i. dresses that have slightly full-cut bodices that nip in at the waist with same color belt
j. pleated or draped skirts
k. "petite" proportioned dresses and other garments
l. simple straight-leg pants (no cuff); cuffs tend to cut height
m. delicate jewelry
n. medium to small prints
o. soft-line double knits, wools; medium to heavy cottons, taffetas, velvets, tweeds
p. medium to light natural-tone stockings
q. medium- to high-heel shoes (not heavy or bulky)

AVERAGE HEIGHT BUT TOO THIN

The average height—too thin figure can also be a fun problem to solve. You can wear clothing that so many women can't. Keep in mind only that you shouldn't wear clothing too tight, and that short skirts (as opposed to floor length) should not be exceedingly full as your legs will appear thinner. The romantic look is for you if you like it.

The first picture shows the average height—too thin figure as it really is.

The second picture shows the same figure dressed incorrectly. In trying to compensate for her thinness, this woman has chosen clothes that give her an unbalanced, and therefore unattractive look.

The third picture shows what can be done to give the illusion of a heavier figure.

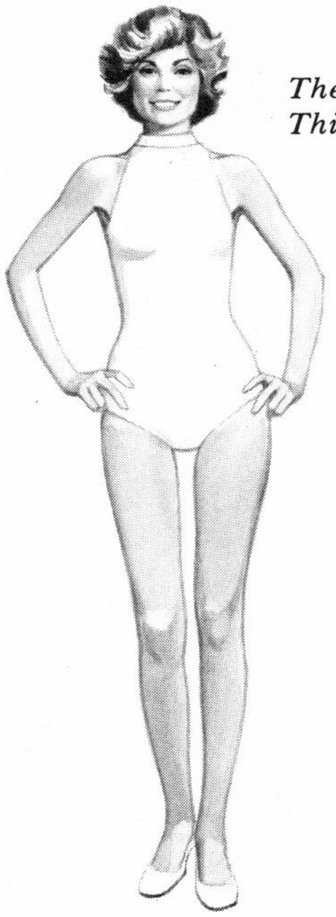

The Average Height, Thin Figure

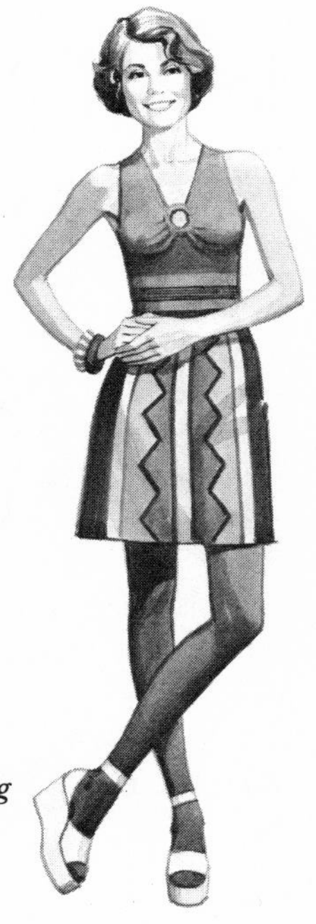

dressed wrong

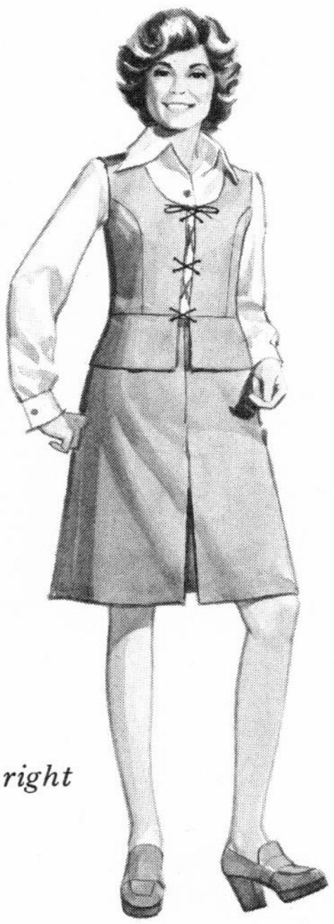

dressed right

AVOID:

a. large or bulky jewelry
b. overly tight or skimpy garments
c. vertical stripes or patterns
d. sleeveless dresses, unless the shoulder seam is cut in considerably

e. deep-cut dresses or blouses
f. any garments that are overpowering: big capes and coats, very bulky sweaters, big hats
g. pants with no pockets
h. dark stockings
i. heavy or cumbersome shoes or boots

DO WEAR:

a. hair soft and not too short
b. minimal amount of jewelry—and keep it on the delicate side
c. scarves on neck or blouse if desired
d. garments with simple fullness around bust and hips; make sure the bottom of a street-length skirt is not overly full as this will make your legs appear thinner
e. straight-type skirt or dress if it is of a heavier-type fabric and a medium-size fabric design
f. light solid colors to give illusion of being heavier
g. horizontal lines and design to give width to the figure
h. clothes that are cut for smaller slimmer proportions (such as Junior sizes)
i. overblouse or layered look (vest or sweater over blouse, etc.)
j. soft-look dresses in small-scale prints
k. hemline just touching or covering your knee (but not calf)
l. pants and skirts with pockets
m. medium- to light-tone stockings
n. shoes that are not heavy or clunky-looking
o. boots that reach up to your skirt hemline; or skirt should overlap top of boots

TALL AND TOO THIN

In dressing to give the illusion of added pounds and less height, remember these basic rules: never wear your clothes too tight, too loose, or baggy. They will only make you appear thinner. A low-heeled shoe, a simple hairstyle, and the right choice of fabric design will give you less height. You can enjoy the dramatic look. Bright colors, large patterns, vivid contrasts—these are all for you.

The first picture shows the tall and thin figure as it really is.

The second picture shows the same figure dressed incorrectly, with the figure unbalanced.

The third picture shows the result of the proper choice of clothing style, fabrics, hairstyle, and accessories.

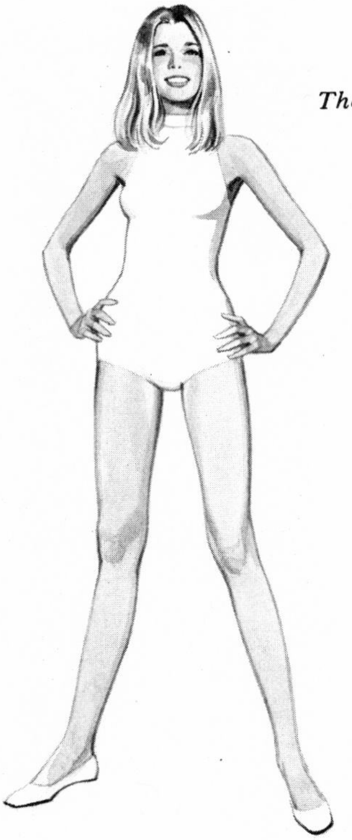

The Tall, Thin Figure

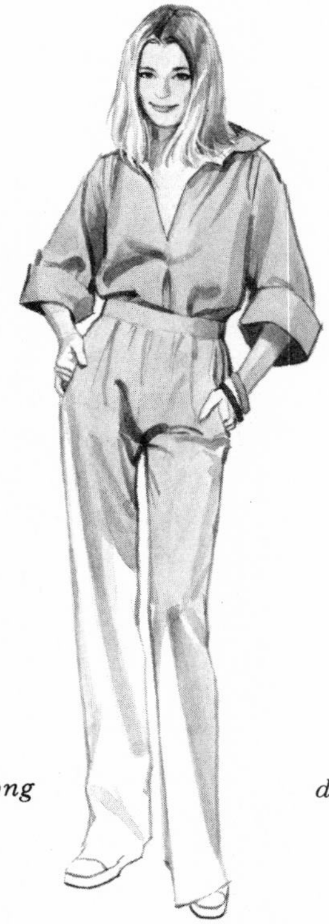

dressed wrong

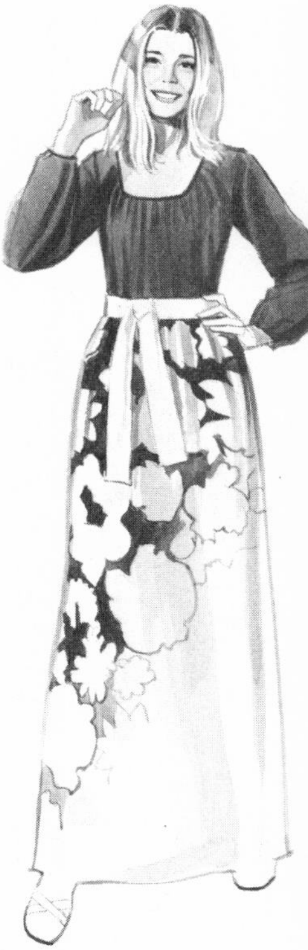

dressed right

AVOID:

a. bouffant hairstyles (keep it soft and simple)
b. garments overly tight or skimpy; clingy fabrics
c. overly full garments
d. vertical stripes or patterns
e. dark solid colors
f. one-piece dress with no belt
g. sleeveless dresses, unless the shoulder seam is cut in considerably
h. deep-cut dresses or blouses
i. hems above the knee; clothing that is too short for the arms or legs
j. pants with no pockets
k. heavy or clunky-looking shoes

DO WEAR:

a. hair that is not too short, worn down to soften total look (at least to middle of neck, but to shoulders if possible)
b. scarves on neck or blouse, when possible
c. jewelry that is medium size
d. soft long-sleeved blouse, when possible
e. bulky sweaters reaching past your waistline
f. the layered look—one sweater or vest over a blouse, when possible
g. white or light solid colors to give the illusion of being heavier
h. medium- to large-scale fabric designs
i. horizontal fabric design and detailing
j. simple fullness around bust and hips (not *overly* full—too many gathers will make your legs and body appear thinner)
k. straight-type skirt or dress if it is of a fairly heavy fabric and a medium-size design (like suits or simple one-piece dresses)
l. different colored skirt (or pants) and blouse to break your height
m. broken lines at waist—easily achieved by wearing a wide belt or sash
n. pants and skirts with pockets—it "adds weight"
o. cuffed pants to cut length
p. medium to light natural-tone stockings
q. medium- to low-heeled shoes; make sure slacks and long dresses touch the tops of the shoes. Pants and dresses that are too short will only make you appear taller and awkward. Simple, classic, graceful shoe styles are the most flattering

Chapter Seven

THE VITAL FUNCTION OF UNDERGARMENTS-WHAT'S BEST FOR YOU

Undergarments have truly been given the most appropriate name possible: "foundation"! If you have a figure problem, foundations are the very beginning of molding the body image you want. They can make or break your illusion.

The correct undergarments can go a long way toward giving you the illusion of a more perfect figure. The wrong undergarments can ruin a perfectly beautiful look. They will not only fail to enhance your figure, but they can make you look downright sloppy—or silly.

There are no two figures really alike. But with balance and a little figure illusion, almost every type of figure can be made to look terrific. There are so many new garments being designed today that you should ask "What's new?" each time you shop for undergarments.

If you have never been fitted by an expert and feel you need this help, the first step is to find a lingerie shop that is well stocked and has expert sales help available. A large department store or a lingerie boutique would be ideal.

After your first visit to a reputable store, they will know your needs and be able to help you more quickly and efficiently the next time you visit them. By reading this chapter, you will become acquainted with the basic types of undergarments and be able to ask for the things most appropriate for you. Keep trying on garments until you find what is most comfortable, most becoming, and most effective in coping with your particular problem.

If you are buying undergarments to wear with a specific outfit, take that outfit with you or wear it, if possible. There is no surer way to save yourself a trip to the store to return unsuitable merchandise.

When looking for an expert in this field to collaborate on this chapter with us, we were fortunate to find Ben Schwartz of Schwartz Lingerie in Chicago. Mr. Schwartz stated that never before in his career had the manufacturers been producing such a wide range of practical and beautiful garments. To give an idea of how much choice you actually have nowadays, we will discuss below the types of undergarments made for different parts of the body.

BUST

It is difficult to exaggerate the importance of your bustline in the total body image you are presenting to the world. The same bust can take on different shapes and sizes, and create different impressions, depending upon the type of brassiere worn. A store that has a wide range of types will give you the opportunity to see which ones do the most for you.

Even if you have no specific bust problem, the choice of a bust foundation garment is a very important element in your figure illusion, and deserves more than casual and purely fashion-minded attention.

To find a brassiere with exactly the right look and fit you may have to try on a lot of different styles by different manufacturers, but it is well worth the effort to find the most flattering style for you. Unless you are buying a bra to wear with a specific garment or outfit—in which case, as we suggested, take it along with you to your fitting sessions—it is best to try on a bra under a soft blouse or top. That way you can see exactly how the bra shapes you, and whether it is to your best advantage. Remember that the objective is to look as if it's you and only you under that blouse. The best look is the most natural one, where you don't notice the bra (one reason that proper fit is so important—to avoid the little signs that disrupt a figure illusion and make the things creating that illusion all too obvious). A too-large cup will create "hollow tips" or, if too small, "bumps" or bulges at the top or sides of the bra. A bra that is too tight will create bulges and creases. There will be a line of demarcation—an indentation—where the elastic digs into the body, and then a bulge on either side.

Bra straps should not be so tight that they create an indentation on the shoulder, nor so loose that they drop out of a sleeve. Be sure you are wearing a low-cut bra for styles that are scoop neck or lower. Bra straps should never show when you wear a short-sleeve or sleeveless top.

To determine your proper cup size, measure your chest just below the bust. Then measure your bust, without a bra, at the fullest point (usually approximately at the nipples).

If the difference in measurement is 1 inch, your cup size is A. If it is 2 inches, your cup size is B. If it is 3 inches, your cup size is C, and if 4 inches, your cup size is D. (Larger sizes than D usually require special fitting, preferably by a knowledgeable lingerie shop or department.) For example, if your chest (or "rib cage") is 34 inches, and your bust 36, your bra size is 34B.

If the difference in measurement between chest and bust falls between 2 and 3 inches, for instance, try on both the B and C cups, and judge how the two different sizes feel and look on you. A little loose is generally preferable to a little tight (and the resulting binding or "slightly pushed out" effect).

Don't think you're the only one with a bust problem—rare is the woman who hasn't, at some point in her life, anguished over and mentally reshaped her bustline. Just because the bustline is so common a problem, bust undergarments, especially in recent years, have had the benefit of a lot of expert attention. There is a better designed, more glamorous, ingeniously flattering, and wider array of "special" bras available today than ever before.

The following are the main types available for specific bust-problem needs.

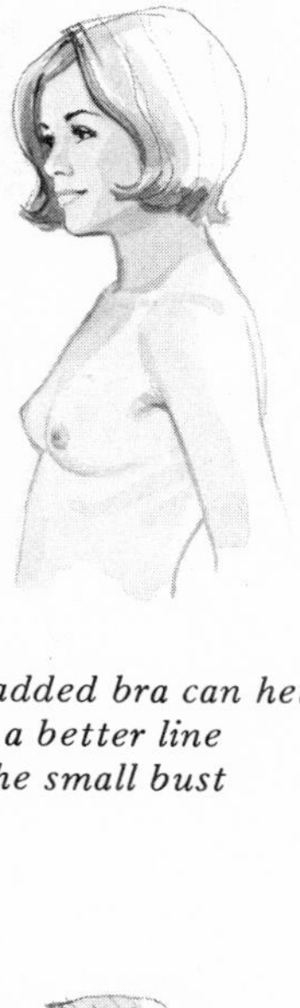

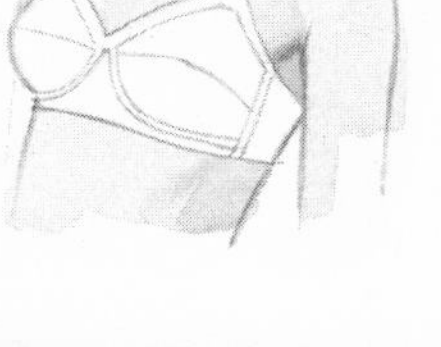

A padded bra can help give a better line to the small bust

Bust Too Small

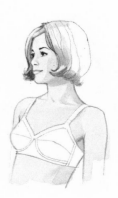

a. *padded bra*—entire cup moderately to heavily padded (at least ¼-inch, some even more). This type of bra is bought in the size you would have taken in an unpadded bra. A regular padded bra won't give cleavage, and must be chosen with care to avoid a "pointed," seamed, or otherwise unnatural look. Such a bra must also be chosen and fitted with even more care than a regular bra. Some discretion must be used in wearing padded bras under highly clingy or low-cut garments. It is best to try the bra on beneath a soft blouse (or the specific garment you intend to wear it with) so you can judge the total effect—the line and fullness it gives you

b. *semi-padded*—entire cup moderately to lightly padded, with a soft lining. This bra is for the woman with less of a problem in this area, who wants a fuller, more rounded look (or who simply feels more comfortable and confident with a more natural look)

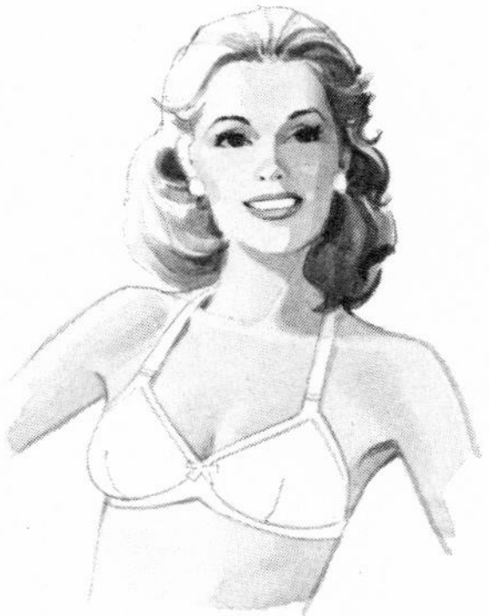

A softly lined contour bra will subtly enhance the natural curves of the small-to-medium bust

c. *contour bra*—entire cup lined with a soft lining; this bra is not padded, but has just enough soft lining to make a uniform shape and subtly enhance the natural curves

d. *push-up bra*—available in regular and strapless styles. Padding or lining at lower part of the cup "pushes up" the available flesh to create a lusher look, cleavage for low-cut tops and garments

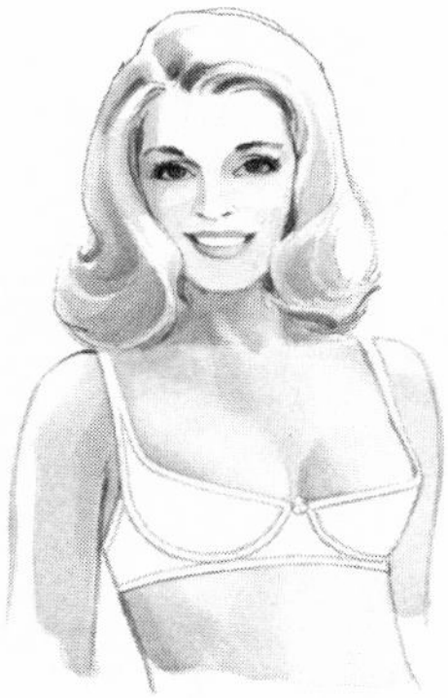

A push-up bra is flattering for the small-to-medium bust (and for the average bust with low-cut garment styles)

e. *foam half-cups*—can be purchased separately and positioned in a bra to create a push-up effect. These half-cups can be bought at lingerie stores and specialty shops

Full separate cups can also be bought to wear with a bra you already own. Both the full and half separate cups must be fitted carefully for it is possible for them to work their way up and out of position. (How's that for shattering an illusion?)

Here are a few "bosom-enhancing" tricks that models use:

1. For instant push-up effect in a jiffy, stuff "evenly crumpled" tissue into your bra under the bust, and on the sides, and your bust will be pushed up and to the center for cleavage.

2. To create (or enhance) the effect of cleavage line, use a brown eye shadow or eyebrow pencil to make a muted, smudged ½-inch-wide line at the spot where your cleavage should be.
3. If you are going braless and don't want to feel self-conscious (or let it be too obvious that you are not wearing a bra) put Band-Aids over your nipples. You can also tape up your breasts for a more secure braless look. (This will also give you more cleavage for a low-cut neckline.) Holding your breasts up, run the tape from right under one arm to under the other. How wide an adhesive tape you need will depend on how full you are.

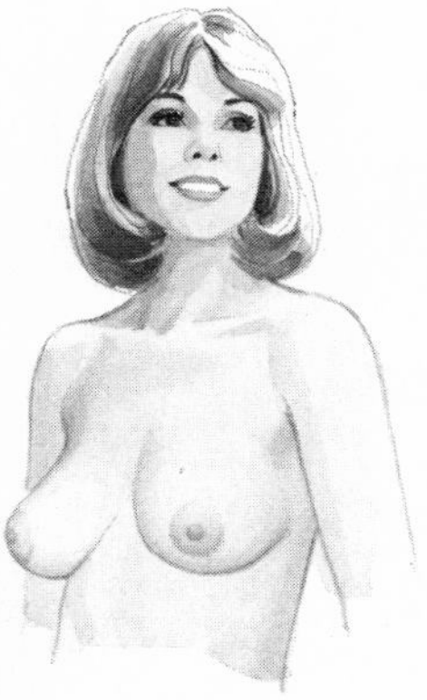

Bust Too Large

a. "minimizer"—for the woman with a very large bust; moves flesh around to a more desirable position, to the side or front, depending on the individual woman's needs, balancing the flesh on the top part of the body better

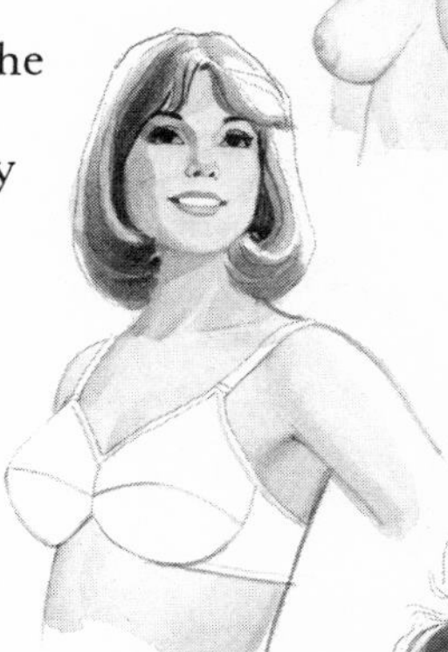

A minimizer is helpful for the Bust Too Large

b. boned bra—built-in (usually plastic) bones give extra support for the heavy bust
c. underwire bra—gives more support with covered wiring under the breast. Available strapless or with straps

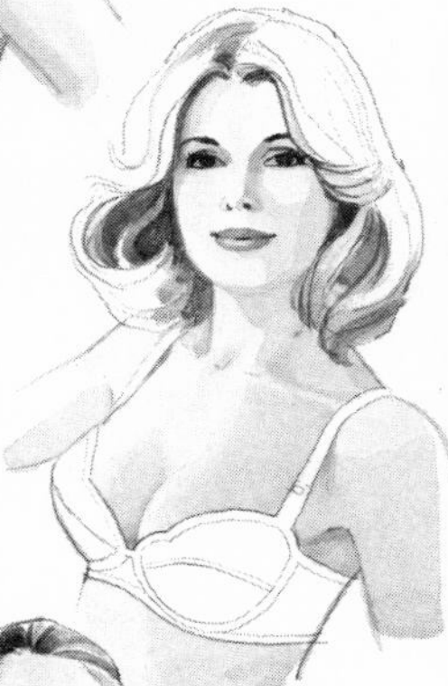

An underwire bra

Note: If a bra bone is cutting into your flesh, bend the bone or wire to form a more open circle, until it feels comfortable.

Bras for the Heavy Figure

a. full-cut—gives full support all over. Covers the entire bust, has wider straps, and a very wide band around the back. Usually cut higher underneath the arm and higher in the back. Good for fleshy backs.

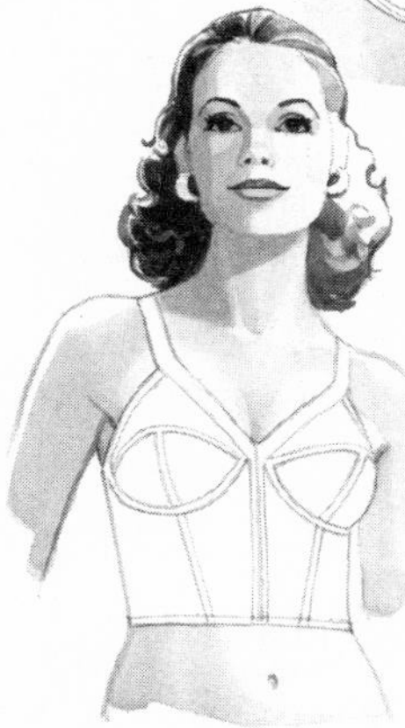

A waist-length or "short-length" bra

b. "longline" bras are available in a variety of lengths, from those with a ½-inch control band below the bust, to waist-length styles that help flatten out midriff bulges. There are even styles which extend a few inches beyond the waist, to insure a smooth line to the waist and below, and help control hips and stomach.

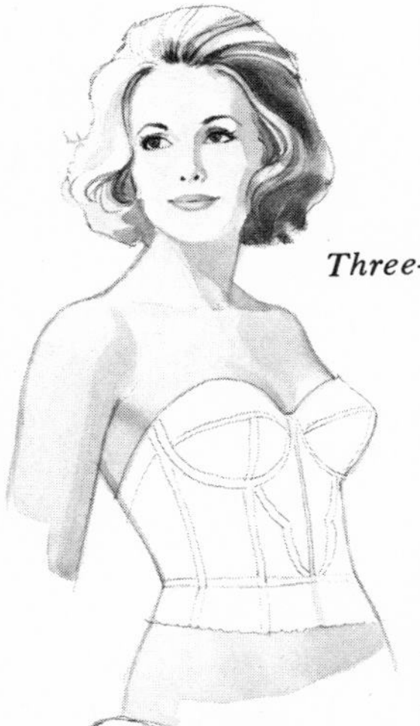

Three-quarter length or longline bra

c. bra-slip—a combination garment of elasticized firm fabric (and often bones) down to the waist, with a regular slip below. Gives a smooth line from top to bottom and helps smooth out midriff bulge

For the Woman With Prosthetic Bra Needs

A prosthesis bra is a special bra for women who have had surgery in which one or both breasts were removed. The bra has an opening built in so that a pocket of silicone gel or individually shaped foam padding can be inserted to make the breast look normal and natural. The American Cancer Society has listings of shops that sell these individually fitted special bras.

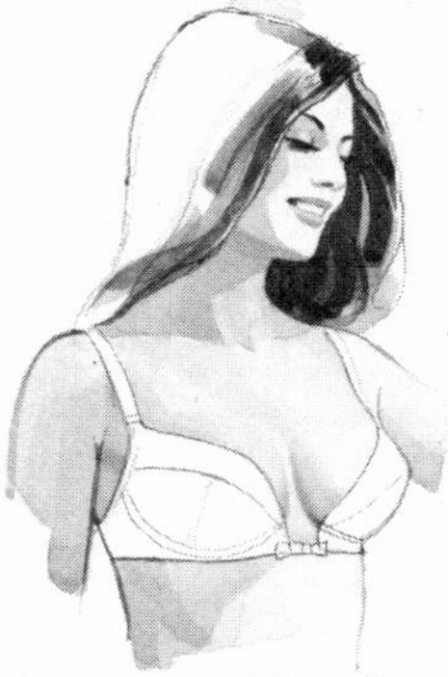

The plunge bra

Bras for Special Fashion Needs

a. low-cut bra—supports the under part of the breast, leaving the top part exposed for uniformly low-cut garments
b. plunge bra—low cut in the center, for deep plunging necklines
c. décolletage bra—low cut, shoulder straps on edge of shoulders—for scoop-neck and low-cut garments
d. push-up bra—padding in lower part of cups pushes up breasts for a fuller look in low-cut garments
e. halter or convertible—crisscross straps, detachable. Some can be worn as many as five different ways. (Straps can get very close to neck for halter garments)
f. strapless bras—designed to support the bust without the use of straps, often incorporating a push-up feature. Be sure the dress or top you are planning to wear a strapless with will accommodate the extra fullness without looking strained or artificial. Strapless and bandeau bras are very similar, except that the bandeau (also known as

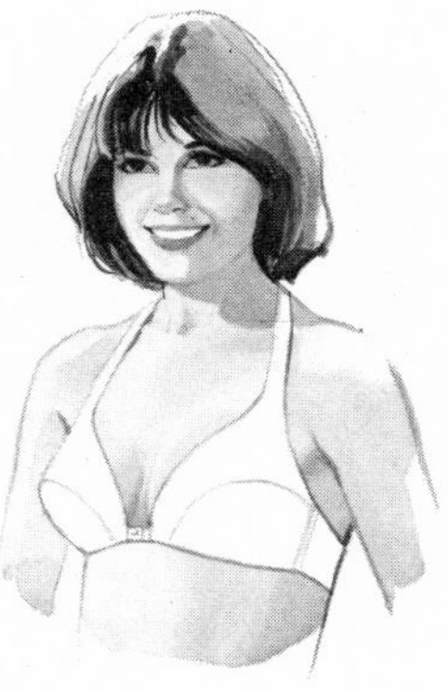

Halter bra

the binder, or tube) does not have a wire under the breast. The strapless longline can go to the waist or to the hip, gives a smooth line from the bust to the bottom of the bra, and cinches the waist. Make sure, when you are trying on a strapless, that it stays up properly and feels secure (or you can be sure it won't when you wear it outside)

g. front-hook bra—hooks in front, leaves flat, smooth line in back
h. "nude" or "nearly nude" bra—seamless, often flesh-colored bra of a thin, stretch, often knitted fabric that supports, but gives the illusion of no bra
i. sweater bra—seamless cup, smooth line with no wrinkles or seams. Available in contour, molded, and padded styles
j. cocktail bra—glues on to skin, for use under a dress or other garment with a lot of exposure. Two types: 1. push-up (lifts or molds)—only for small to average, covers half the breast. 2. Glue-on that covers the whole bust—for dress that might be sideless, backless, but has all of breast covered

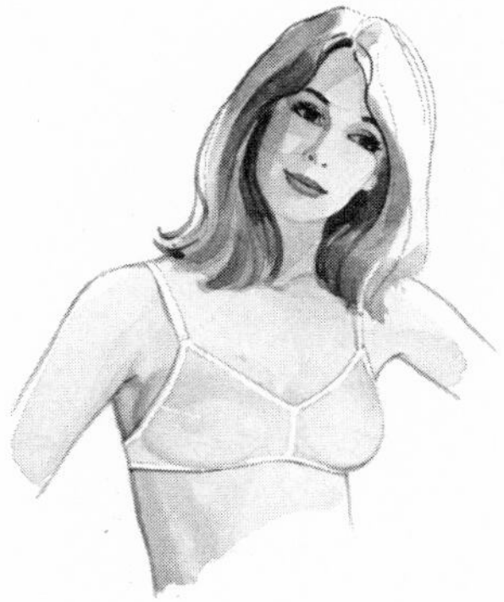

The seamless-cup sweater bra

HIPS, STOMACH, AND DERRIERE

The basic function of what used to be called a girdle is to firm too-full hips, stomach, and derriere; to take inches off these areas and in general improve the line of the body under garments.

Though firm-control foundation garments have fallen into disfavor in some quarters in recent years, they are still a highly effective "short-term" way to improve appearance and posture (and there are even types available now that will reduce in size, as you reduce).

The girdle industry has improved its product tremendously—you don't have to be laden down with heavy, hot, thick, zippered garments anymore. The new lightweight lines are just as effective as the older ones, and come in a much greater range of styles, but it is hard for some women to break long-standing habits. The lightweight garments have the same control and quality and are easier to put on and more comfortable to wear. If you need a girdle, try the lightweight type and see if it doesn't improve your comfort.

Buttocks Too Wide and Too Large, Stomach Too Full

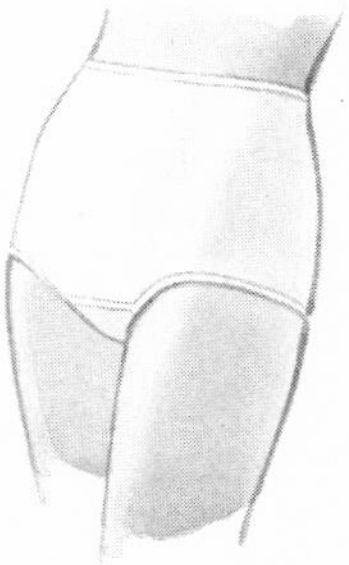

Lightly elasticized panty brief

a. lightly elasticized panty brief or bikini—great for minimal stomach or hip control, for the woman with a minor problem in these areas
b. panty girdle—lightweight elasticized control garment, often with attached garters, that covers more area than a panty brief would. Light overall firming of stomach and buttocks
c. the garter belt—the type useful for stomach control is wider, extending from waist to at least midstomach. For women who don't wear panty-hose, the "control" garter belt can give a more confident feeling, and is more comfortable than the narrow styles of garter belt. (Narrow styles of garter belt are usually worn purely for "fashion" purposes; these come in satin, lace, and cotton, and may cut across the stomach at a point that calls attention to the stomach in an unflattering way)
d. panty stockings, "tummy control" stockings, support hose—come with a built-in elasticized brief (some also have elasticized thighs); give mild firmness and control of the lower body. (For the "frequent runner," the tummy control stockings have the disadvantage that a run in the stocking part necessitates discarding the entire panty stocking, and of course these are more costly than regular panty-hose)
e. regular girdle—firmly elasticized garment, usually with stronger control panels in front, back, and/or sides. Comes in heavy, medium, and lightweight, and short, average, and long lengths. Be sure the flesh does not bulge at the legs or stomach where the garment stops. If this happens it means that the girdle is too small or in some other way not the right fit for you. We cannot overemphasize the fact that you must take the time to try on garments until you find the right one for you. Don't be satisfied with less than perfect fit!

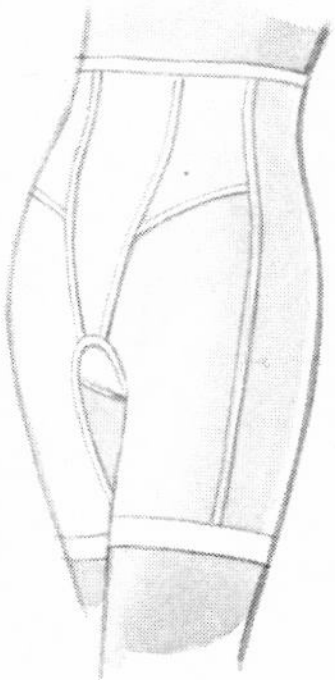

Strong-control panty girdle

FOR OVERALL CONTROL AND SLIMMING

a. The lightweight bodysuits can be worn under very sheer, clingy fabrics that need a smooth, continuous, uniform line from the shoulders to the hips or legs. These bodysuits (or body stockings) are also good for the figure that is a little too full or loose—they hold the body firm but keep it soft-looking

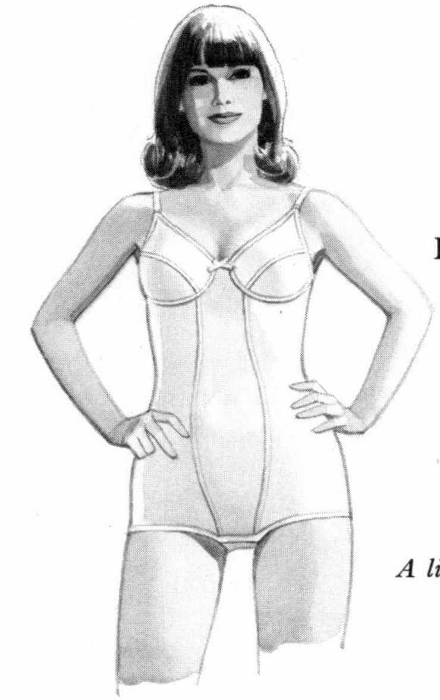

A lightweight bodysuit

b. The heavier bodysuits can be used for a smooth line under evening dresses or special outfits that might show the outline of other undergarments. They have plastic stays and, often, control panels that hold the body in from the bust down to the buttocks

Both the lightweight and the heavier bodysuits come in mid-thigh and top-of-the-thigh lengths. Both types are available in pullover or zippered styles (be sure the zipper is flat enough not to show), usually with a snap-off crotch. The heavier bodysuits usually have garters, to be worn with stockings, and these help keep a girdle or bodysuit in place.

Be sure that you choose the bodysuit length that covers the largest part of your problem, if you have heavy legs, or a bulge will be inevitable at the "garter line."

For Waistline Slimming

All types of girdles have high waists for those who need them (some have as much as a 4-inch band). If the store at which you are shopping doesn't have the needed width of band, go to another store, or to a professional seamstress who can sew a band on for you.

a. the longline bra mentioned earlier pulls the waist in
b. the waist-cinch, usually 6 inches wide, comes in waist sizes of small, medium, and large. This can be worn for special effects, especially in the evening with full-skirted dresses

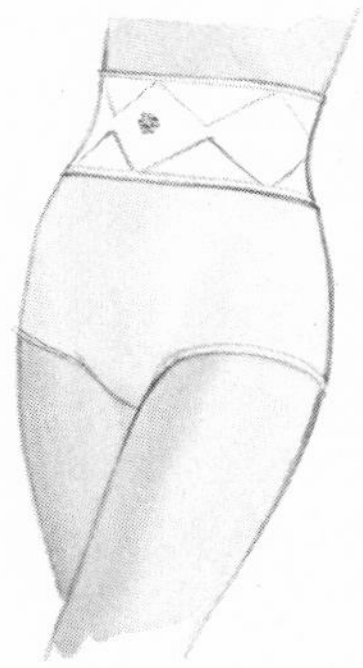

Waist-cinch

Note: When trying on waist-length bras and other waist slimmers, be sure that there are no bulges created at the top or bottom of the garment; if such bulges occur, try the next size.

Heavy Thighs

a. panty girdles have legs in long and short lengths. Choose the length that does not leave a bulge at the bottom
b. slack girdles go from the waist to the calf, leaving no creases or lines between waist and calf on slacks
c. the control stockings mentioned under "Buttocks Too Wide" give some degree of control of heavy thighs

Buttocks Blending Into Legs (lack of a definite inward curve under the derriere)

"Molded backside"—soft panties, briefs, and girdles that are constructed by a method of sewing the seat of the garment so that it allows the rounded part of the buttocks to be natural, and give slightly firmer support underneath. They give separation between the buttocks and the legs and also stay in place under the buttocks, never riding up.

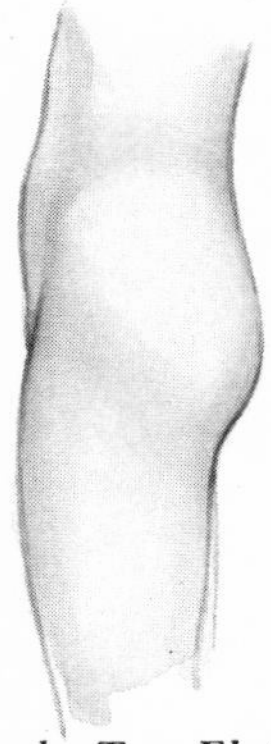

Buttocks Too Flat—before

Buttocks Much Too Thin or Abnormal

Padded hip girdles and padded buttocks girdles are products that are not in as great a demand as the ones mentioned above, but they are available. Frederick's of Hollywood is among the manufacturers. There are not many women who are thin enough to need these, but they may be especially helpful to women who are irregularly formed either congenitally or through accidents, operations, or illnesses that may cause loss of flesh in these areas.

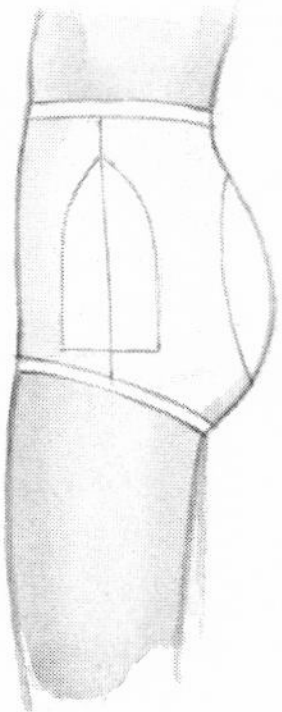

With specially padded girdle

SLIPS

Slips are not the indispensable undergarment they once were, but there are times when a slip is called for to give your outfit a more unified line or to make the garment you are wearing opaque and keep it in the realm of good taste. Slips can also help disguise the lines of bra and panties, as well as help to prevent certain knit or synthetic fabrics from clinging too much.

Full slips: if a dress is translucent, a full slip can help give a finished look (it is acceptable for some evening dresses to be slightly translucent).

A half-slip is worn to prevent skirts from appearing too translucent. Such slips usually have elasticized waistbands—be sure you get a proper fit to prevent the slip from riding or rolling up onto the elastic. If you are heavy (or heavy-hipped), avoid very full, bulky fabrics, thick with decoration.

The thin or small-busted woman can gain some advantage from shirred-top and shaped-bodice styles; the large-busted or heavy woman should stay away from these.

Both the full and the half-slip should be long enough to touch the top of the hem of the garment they are worn beneath. A slip should never show or hang beneath the hem. Too full a slip, by adding excess fabric under a skirt, can make heavy (or any) hips look fuller. A slip of too dark a color or pattern beneath a light-colored garment will create distracting or disturbing effects.

Pettipants are in reality a form of short slip that can simultaneously serve as underpants. They can be chosen to leave a smooth line on the leg or to have lace and ruffles, meant to show under a very short outfit. If a skirt is translucent, choose a half slip, rather than pettipants.

Petticoats or crinolines are still occasionally called for to help fill out a special look (for example, a peasant look or a country square-dance costume). Obviously the generally heavy woman, the woman with a heavy waist or heavy hips, and the woman with thin legs—if it is a short crinoline—must be very wary of this style.

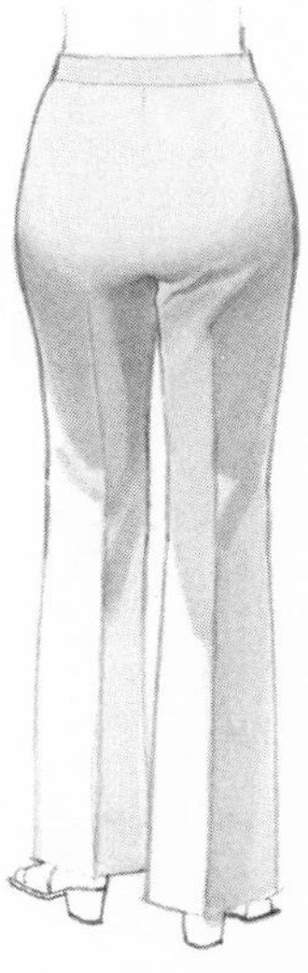

Right

A NOTE ON UNDERPANTS

When wearing slacks (especially tight slacks) be sure to wear panties that do not ride up the buttocks. It's not half as becoming (or sexy) a sight as that of *no* panty line. Also make sure they are not bulky or too tight (try a size larger), causing a ridge to show above or below the panty line. There is a regular panty with a seam up the middle of the back that is designed in such a way that it hugs and never creeps up. Creeping is less likely to happen with panties that have elastic at the legholes.

Another "under-wear" oversight that has a tendency to wreak havoc with figure illusion is the matter of tucking in tops. Too often tops worn "in" carelessly (with pants and skirts) add bulk to the waist and hip line and create disrupting, unsightly lumps and bulges.

Pay attention to the length of the "tails" or bottom hem of a top or blouse—soft, light-fabric tails can safely be longer than bulky fabrics, but in all cases take care that there is not a

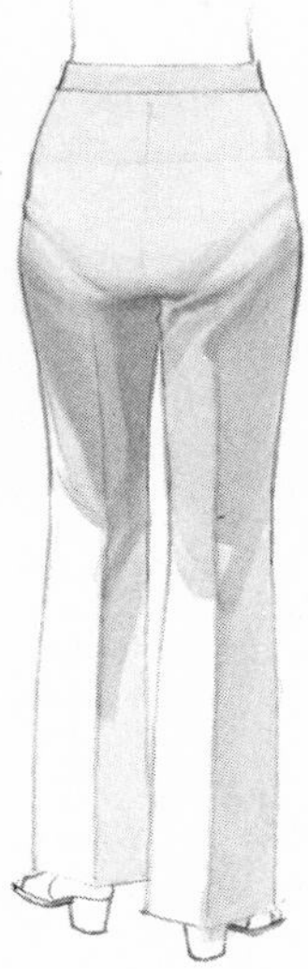

Wrong

bulky hem and (especially if you are heavy) that it does not hit the widest part of the hips (it will usually be semi-visible, even under clothing).

Simply cramming all the "overlap" under your panties, panty girdle, etc. does not solve the problem (and indeed may worsen it). It may well be worthwhile to shorten tails or total length of heavy fabric tops you intend to wear "in" and tailor sides (and in some cases dart the front of) blouses to cut down on the amount of excess fabric that must be disposed of when you tuck in a shirt or blouse. Bulky decorative details that extend beyond the visible waistline also bear scrutiny. Remember in such tailoring to *cut away,* not merely fold over, the excess fabric.

Now that you have an idea of the world of expertly designed "helpers" at your disposal, don't hesitate to go to the lingerie department and ask to try on as many types as you like. It's very important to be open-minded. Don't say no to a style unless you have actually tried it on. That's the *only* way to tell.

Chapter Eight

HOW ACCESSORIES CAN IMPROVE YOUR FIGURE

Accessories must be chosen carefully. For they are not just worn to give your *outfit* a spark or a special look—they should be worn first and foremost to give *you* a better total look, to heighten and complete your illusion of a perfectly proportioned figure. And most accessories do affect your total image for better or worse. Find yourself below and select your accessories so that the effect is definitely for the better.

BELTS

Belts can be worn to make waistlines appear smaller, higher, or lower. They can be worn to break a tall body-line, to make the person appear shorter, and, worn slightly differently, they can make a short, or short-waisted woman took taller.

A wide belt makes your waist appear higher. A narrow belt can be worn at the bottom of the waistline to give the appearance of a longer torso. A long-waisted person can wear two narrow belts, one above the other, to make the waist appear higher.

A belt worn on the hips with hip hugger pants or hip hugger skirts will make the short-waisted and long-legged combination appear more balanced by giving the illusion of shorter legs and a longer torso. A short person should not wear a belt—unless it's the same color as the dress—because it cuts her height even more. Stay away from novelty belts of any kind unless they are to be worn with a very simple outfit. They are often busy, call too much attention to themselves, and can negate the carefully balanced overall image you are trying to create.

When checking yourself in your full-length mirror, if there is any question about whether the belt *adds* to your overall image, it should probably be removed. Belts should only be worn when they give a definite *plus* to your total image.

If you are wearing a belt just to hold up a skirt, or to bring in your waistline an inch or two, shame on you! Take the garment off and sew the waistline to fit. Belts are an accessory that can be overdone.

BOOTS

These are an accessory to be approached with caution, since the higher boots especially "break" the line of a leg and can disrupt the total illusion you are trying to create. Boots should be worn only with the sporty look—though within that look they can be worn with pants, skirts, or dresses.

In general, the heavy-legged woman should stay away from boots. The extra bulk, and break in the legline, are something else she can do without.

A thin-legged woman may gain some advantage from judiciously selected "higher" styles of boot that meet or go higher than the hem of the skirt or dress they are worn with. In general, boots look more appealing on the tall or medium-tall woman; boots on a short woman can make her appear even shorter.

All figure types should avoid highly decorated, two-tone, or brightly colored boots as they call too much attention to themselves and create a "costume" effect.

Short (such as ankle-high) boots should usually be worn only under pants. Almost any woman is bound to look awkward or ill-proportioned with a garment that shows leg (stockinged or otherwise) above short boots.

High boots can be worn over your pants but make sure the pants are not too full in the leg or the look will be sloppy. Even high boots can be worn under pants but, of course, this is an absolute no-no for the heavy-legged woman.

Skirts—boots should be worn with sporty skirts only; they do not go well with soft or dressy materials. If you are wearing a skirt below the knee, the bottom of the skirt should overlap the top of the boots. If you are wearing a skirt above the knee, don't wear boots—wear shoes instead, or you may be taken for a drum majorette.

Dresses—follow the same rules as for skirts.

COATS AND RAINCOATS

Outerwear should be chosen carefully to make sure it, too, becomes your figure. The wrong type of overcoat can—like a poorly chosen dress or suit—make you appear heavier, shorter, or taller than you really are and want to look.

Here are the rules:

If you are too tall, wear a belted coat to cut your height. Wear medium to dark solid colors. Wear hems 1 or 2 inches below the knee.

If you are tall and too thin, wear a double-breasted coat. The fur-trimmed collar is also good for you.

If you are too short-waisted, wear unbelted coats (unless you are over 5′8″, and then you can "fake" a longer waist with the belted look) to camouflage your short waist.

If you must wear a belted coat, wear a *thin* belt, slightly below your real waistline.

If you have narrow shoulders and broad hips, wear soft shoulder-padded coats to balance your hips, or a simple A-line coat. Avoid pockets at hip level.

If you have narrow hips and broad shoulders, wear soft-shouldered coats with pockets at hip level, and single-breasted jackets.

If you have small hips and a large chest or bust, wear coats with a bit of flair at the bottom. Single-breasted coats are best for you, with simple lines and designs on the top of the coat. Avoid belts unless worn loose if you are tall.

If you have a flat chest and large hips, wear double-breasted coats, scarves at your neck, and avoid any tight-fitting-bodice coat styles.

If you are too heavy in general, wear medium to dark colors, single-breasted coats, and A-line rather than gathered-type coats.

If you are too thin in general, wear a fitted-type coat one size larger than your normal size. Wear light and bright colors to give the illusion of being heavier, and wear a scarf to soften your look.

GLASSES

Glasses are usually not an accessory that people have a choice about wearing. But they can serve not only the function of improving your eyesight but, if correctly selected, they can also enhance the shape of your face and your total appearance. There are so many frame and lens styles available today that finding the right glasses for you has the potential of being a real glamour experience.

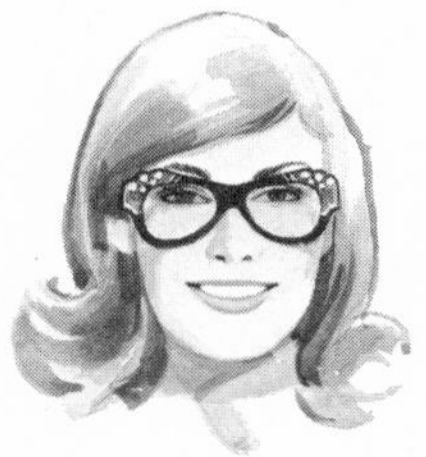

Wrong—Too much decoration, too dark a frame color for her hair color

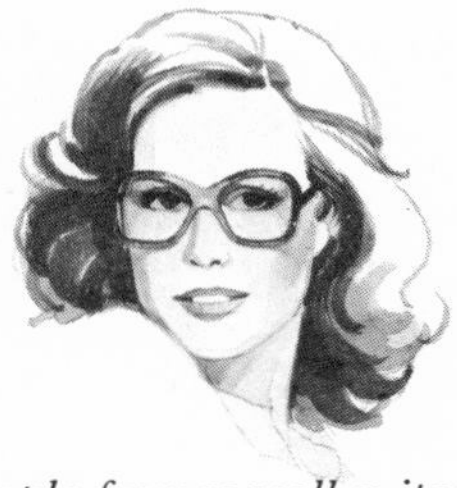

Simple frames well suited to shape and size of the face are best. Glasses should blend in so well that they don't draw attention

Glasses should be selected first on the basis of how they complement your facial structure. When shopping for them, first select two or three pairs that you think look well, remembering in general that glasses should not be so bizarre or flamboyant that people will notice them before seeing the rest of you. They should be part of your total look, blended in so well that they don't draw attention. Before making your final choice, try each pair on in front of a full-length mirror and see what each does for your total appearance from a distance of a few feet. Are the rims too dark or too light? Are the rims too thick? Do they give your face a needed "lift" rather than a harsh or "down" look? Are they too large or too small for your body or head size? (Frames should not extend much beyond the widest point of the cheekbone, viewed from the front.) Very large lenses can usually only be carried by the woman with a large face or head (and even so, choose these with caution). Will they fit into the context of your work and social life?

Frame colors should stay with neutral tones—black, bone, beige, brown, silver, gold, and rimless—unless you are planning to have more than one pair, in which case you should still try to avoid flashy, highly decorated, and novelty color and shape frames. Remember, it is your *face* that you want to be the center of attention. Best color rims for women with dark brown or black hair are: black, brown, silver or gold, and rimless. Best frame colors for women with blonde, red, brown, or light brown hair are: light brown, beige, bone, silver, gold, or rimless. Gray- or silver-haired women look best in silver, rimless, beige, or bone frames.

Prescription and nonprescription lenses are available in a wide variety of tints and shades. Try to stay with brown or gray (or a color your eye doctor recommends), for some tints and shades—especially when worn indoors—are not good for the eyes. And many of them, if you are a person who must wear glasses all the time, or very often, create an unsettling effect on those around you—of colored squares, circles, and so on, around the eyes. Again, it is your face that you want to be the center of attention.

Contact lenses, which can eliminate the need for glasses, may not improve a woman's total appearance in every case because even though they eliminate rims or frames, they may cause tearing of the eyes to some wearers and squinting. If squinting or tearing is your problem, glasses may be better for your general appearance.

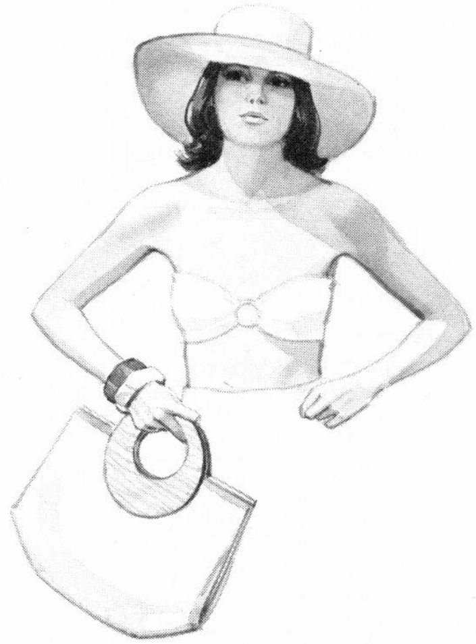

A nice balance in a sporty look for this woman

HANDBAGS

Your handbag is an important part of your total look. It may be more important than you think. Remember that this is an accessory that you wear, or carry, almost constantly; thus it is a genuine part of the "you" you are presenting to the world. The wrong bag can do many negative things to your body illusion.

An oversized bag on a small woman could dwarf her too much.

A tiny bag on a large woman could make the purse look as if it was designed for a child.

A tall woman wearing a very small bag could also accentuate her height.

A thick shoulder bag that hits parallel with a heavy-set woman's hips could make her look even broader. In fact, a very heavy woman should steer clear of shoulder bags. (Carry a bag that is held by the hand or a clutch bag.) But, if it is a "must," then the shoulder bag should be worn above the hips.

A flashy, elaborately decorated bag calls too much attention to itself and is a no-no for daytime wear (though it may be all right if it suits the occasion for evening wear).

A tight-strap shoulder bag worn carelessly with tailored suits or other such clothing can misshape lapels, pull clothing out of shape, and in general detract from the "together" look you are trying to create.

A shoulder strap that cuts diagonally across the body can also wrinkle and distort clothing, and carry the eye directly to itself, again detracting from the total look. It may also emphasize features (such as broad shoulders) that you're trying to disguise.

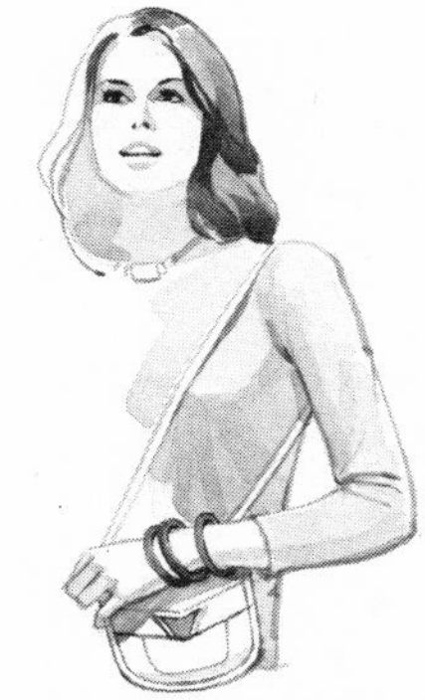

A handbag too small for a tall woman

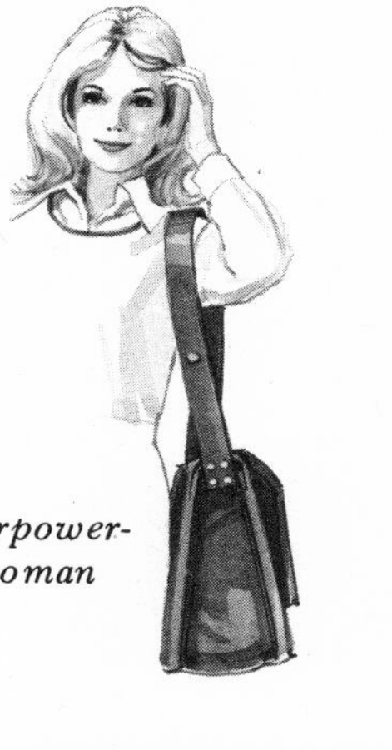

A handbag too overpowering for this small woman

Remember, be careful about the shape, size, and angle where a bag strikes your body. Check your full-length mirror to see the effect from all angles. A small woman should never carry an oversized bag, or a round-shouldered person a shoulder bag. A shoulder (or other long) bag should never hang below the middle of the hips. Also consider that color is important in creating that image you are striving for. Except for special occasions, or as a well-coordinated accessory with special outfits, bag colors should not be bright. If you can only have one or two bags, make them neutral tones, light brown or deep beige, to go with all your wardrobe. Also, prevent your bag from sagging, being misshaped by overstuffing. You will not only look better, but your bags will last much longer.

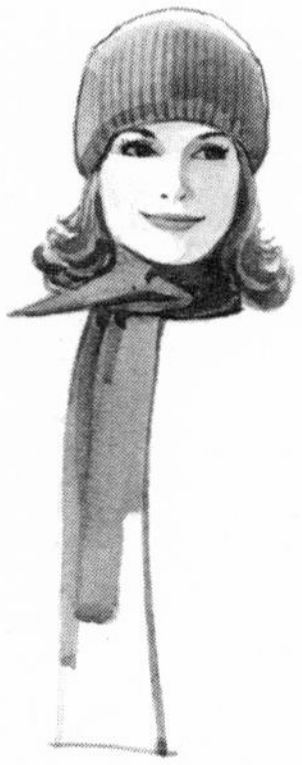

Functional hats have been popular in recent years

HATS

Hats are not the absolute social necessity that they were in previous years. Just a few years ago, a well-dressed woman would not go shopping, to church, or to a wedding without her "crowning accessory." Even though this is not true any longer, a hat can still be an important part of your image when you want a different look.

The hats that seem to be currently popular are ones that serve more functional purposes: sun hats, rain hats, or cold-weather hats—as well as the "just-for-fun" hats. But a hat needs to be more than functional or "fun"; it also needs to balance your total image.

There are some general rules that you can follow when purchasing a hat. First of all, don't be in a rush; take the time to view the hat from all angles in a three-way mirror if possible. Look at it close up and then from several feet away in a full-length mirror. A hat might look just fine on your head when you are seeing it at close range, but it might be a totally different story when you look at it on top of your whole body. (Remember, your full-length mirror is still your first best friend!)

Keep a hat on long enough when trying it on to make sure it fits and is comfortable on your head. Remember that your customary hairdo (or the one you intend to wear the hat with) is a major factor determining whether *you* can wear that particular hat. Make sure that a hat is flattering to your hairstyle, and vice versa.

Another thing that can ruin your confidence in your appearance is wondering if a hat is going to stay on—and proper fit is a large part of the answer. There are some styles (such as very large-brimmed hats) that will be a problem under windy conditions, even if they are the right size, unless they come with a tie or chin strap (or you have mastered the art of hat pinning).

Don't wear a hat as a camouflage for a messy or nonexistent hairdo—odds are that's exactly what it will look like.

Large or heavy women should not wear tiny hats that make the figure appear larger. They should avoid small berets and pillboxes. Medium to large hats would be a better balance with this figure.

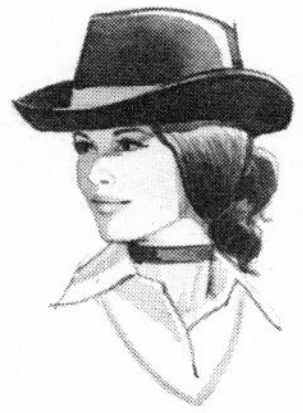

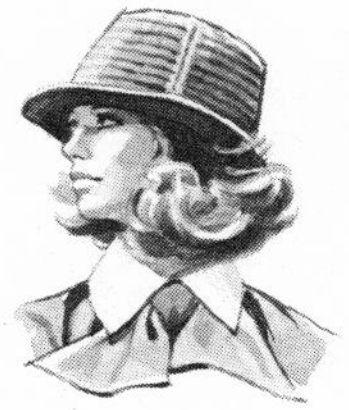

Two well-balanced hat looks

If you have a large head in proportion to your body, you do not want to add a large hat on top of that. If you cannot wear your hair down and full, pull it back and tuck it under a hat to give the illusion of a smaller head and a longer neck.

If you are short and wear your hair down, wear a (not too large) hat with a crown that stands up (even if it has a brim), and you will look taller and slimmer.

If you have a full face, or if you are short and heavy, wear a brim that turns up and away from your face.

If you are tall, wear brims that turn down.

The small woman should stay away from medium- to large-brim hats. She should not wear overly tall hats to give an obviously false illusion—there is a fine line between adding balanced height with a hat and adding a hat much too large or high, resulting in a "stovepipe" appearance. She will only appear smaller from an overall view.

Tall women, if they wear hats at all, should wear medium-large hats and medium-wide brims. High hats add too much height to the tall figure. Also avoid hats that are too tiny.

The woman of average height can wear almost any size hat—just make sure it is not too dominating and that it flatters your face and overall appearance as evidenced by your full-length mirror. You must envision what you will look like to the person coming down the street who sees you as a whole.

JEWELRY

We have stated before that diamonds are a girl's *second* best friend (her mirror being the first!). But not everyone is fortunate enough to have the "real McCoy" when it comes to jewelry. It's good to know that a woman can be extremely well dressed with very little or no jewelry on. Some of the wealthiest women in the world value the simplicity of the understated look, including Jackie Onassis and many others who regularly appear on the "10 Best-Dressed Women" list. And when they wear "sparkling" jewelry, they wear it after 6:00 P.M. Glitter should *always* be saved for that time.

Don't be concerned if you can't keep up with the jet set when it comes to jewels. But remember that even if you can afford to buy real jewels, you need to be concerned with good design. *Keep it simple.* The innate beauty of the gem or metal that you are buying is usually sufficient without getting into gaudy or ostentatious designs and settings. If you are partial to the more highly decorated styles (such as antique jewelry), remember that a "busy" design must be worn with a very simple garment to be effective.

If you are buying costume jewelry, try the following tip: Study good quality jewelry in a fine shop and in top fashion magazines. Try to define what makes it successful, then look at imitation jewelry and try to find these same design principles in it. YOU CAN.

As in the case of the more expensive jewelry, the innate appeal of many of the materials that go into inexpensive jewelry (shell, bone, wood, leather, metals, colored glass, etc.) will usually create a better effect than complex designs and elaborate attempts to "counterfeit" the expensive versions.

Here are some rules to follow when buying jewelry:

Short, thick neck—Stay away from chokers or very short necklaces. Choose pendants, button or short dangle earrings (dangle only for evening), long necklaces, long chains that will draw attention away from your neck.

Heavy arms—Wear a wider bracelet (stay away from the delicate ones) or combine several small ones.

Thin arms—Don't wear bulky bracelets or watches; this makes arms look thinner. Wear more delicate styles and two or three delicate bracelets together, if you wish. Don't go overboard on a thin arm.

Thin neck—Earrings can be dangle- or button-type (not overly large, but more delicate). Chokers or medium-length necklaces are good.

Rings—Large hands can take chunky or larger rings, also two or three thin bands together. A small hand should wear more delicate rings.

The tall woman should wear primarily medium- to large-size jewelry.

The small woman should wear primarily small- to medium-size jewelry.

The large-busted woman should wear medium-size jewelry that "lays flat"—does not stick out on the bust.

The small-busted woman can wear very large jewelry—"bib" necklaces, large pendants and brooches, etc.—to advantage.

The wide-chested woman should wear a necklace extending down almost to the bustline.

The narrow-chested woman should wear the shorter necklace styles.

One last tip about wearing jewelry. Don't wear earrings, necklace, and bracelet all at one time. Don't be overly concerned about jewelry *matching* when you do wear more than one piece as long as the individual items complement each other. Silver and gold can be worn very well together. There is nothing that looks more overdone or unsophisticated than wearing four or five pieces of jewelry at the same time.

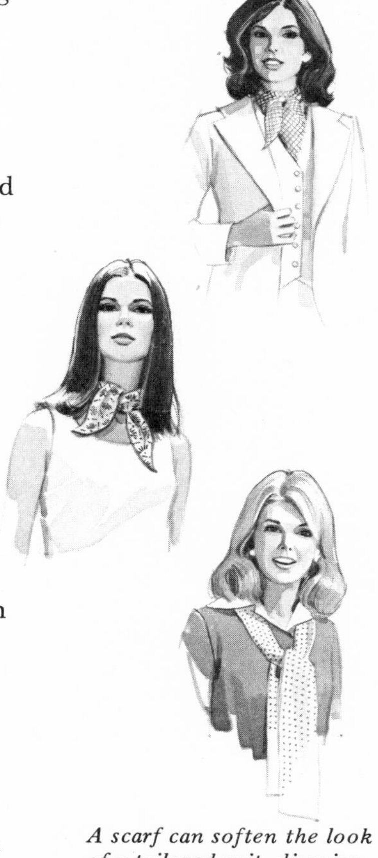

A scarf can soften the look of a tailored suit, disguise a thin or unattractive neck, or a flat chest, small bust

SCARVES

If you've never taken the opportunity to experiment with this silky dash of color, now is the time! A scarf added to an outfit at the right place can give you the perfect finishing touch. It can soften the look of a tailored suit or give you just the dash of color you need with a dark outfit. But there are some figure problems in which a neck scarf should be avoided: *thick necks,* or very short necks, or top-heavyness will only be accentuated by a scarf.

The woman whose neck is too long gains the most corrective benefit from scarves which can reduce the length of a neck considerably (depending on how it is worn) or camouflage a scrawny neck.

Women with flat or bony chests can also benefit from this accessory. How does a scarf around the neck help? The secret is to extend the scarf in a style that falls from the neck to or past the bustline. Scarves can also be used to create the "bowed" or frilly effect on top that we have recommended for the woman with a small bust.

Even a *short or chubby woman* can gain some benefit from a properly worn scarf. She can wear a soft, narrow, long scarf flowing from her neck in an unbroken line down the center of her body, extending past the hips.

SHOES

The first basic rule to follow in selecting shoes is always to choose shoes that are the same tone or darker than the bottom of the dress or slacks you are wearing. They should *never* be lighter! They do not have to be of the same color family, but if you were to take a black and white photo of the shoes and garment, the shoes should appear as dark or darker than the garment.

Following are some other pointers to keep in mind for your particular problem area:

Large women—stay away from shoes so delicate and fragile that they hardly seem able to hold up the body. The thick-strap shoe or standard pump, or even the slingback, is more in balance with this figure.

Feet that are too large or wide—wear a conservative shoe. Wearing two or three colors, a very bright color, or shoes with an eye-catching trim only call attention to large feet. Two shades of the same color (such as medium brown and light brown) are permissible if you feel you would like some variety. Likewise, thick or extreme platform soles and heels only add to the total bulk of large feet.

Unless you have *very* large feet, a higher heel (that is not too thick) and "low-cut" styling, with open toes and heels, will usually help camouflage the large foot.

Short, stubby feet—wear medium-high heels, plain pumps, V-throats, low T-straps, slingback styles. Avoid straps or shoes that rise high on the instep.

Long, slender feet with normal-length legs—wear medium-high heels, sandal straps, high-riding straps, T-straps, asymmetrical straps, and various throatlines, such as the square, round, or off-center. If your foot is extra-long, avoid V-throat lines, sling straps, and high T-straps, which elongate the foot.

Chubby legs or short legs—wear high heels when possible, plain pumps, and d'orsay cuts. Steer clear of wide straps across the instep, low T-straps, shoes with too much ornamentation, two-tone shoes.

Thin legs—wear medium-to-narrow straps and asymmetrical straps, medium-high but not clunky heels. They will make the thin leg look more shapely.

For your total general appearance, make sure the heels of your shoes are not worn down. A run-down heel sends out the wrong message about you: that you don't care enough about your appearance because (maybe) you don't care about or like yourself very much. THIS IS A TURN-OFF! If you don't value yourself enough to keep up your appearance and try to look your best, why should anyone else value you?

One last note about shoes: Be sure that you are not wearing a dressy shoe with the more casual clothes you wear to your daily job. They will not only make your outfit look uncoordinated, but will probably prevent you from being as comfortable as you should be to function well on the job.

No matter what your figure type, never add any accessory without taking a look at yourself in a full-length mirror, standing five or six feet away. The accessory must be seen in balance with your entire body before you can make a valid decision.

Happy accessorizing!

Chapter Nine

YOU AND YOUR SPORTSWEAR

With greater leisure and interest in physical fitness, many women are finding sportswear an increasingly important part of their wardrobes. (And with the new emphasis on women's sports, sportswear has received more design and fashion attention.)

Clothing for many sports calls for a greater degree of figure exposure. Sports clothing, in addition to looking good, must be comfortable in action. It must often serve other practical secondary functions in addition to its "social" one: for instance, it must be durable, sweat-absorbing and, sometimes, cold-resistant. Add to this the fact that many specialized types of clothing must often be purchased by mail or from catalogues—and you see that a greater degree of care must be exercised in the choice of sports clothes for your individual figure.

No matter what sports you choose or what type of outfit you need, there is usually only one style (maybe two) that will do the most for you. Be sure to check under the individual headings elsewhere in this book for your spot or combination problems in general when buying sportswear—the tennis dress or golf skirt that's right for you would be of the same type as already recommended for your figure in a previous chapter. The following are the basic rules to follow in buying outfits for some of the most popular sports.

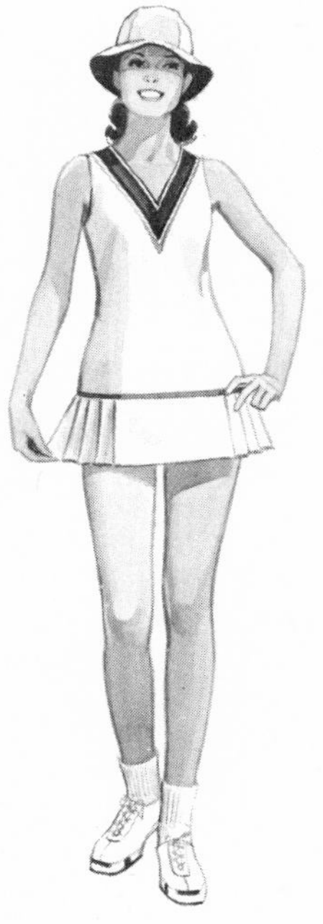

TENNIS WEAR

Great legs—you can wear short tennis dresses.

Legs too heavy—wear them a bit longer, as this gives the illusion of a slimmer leg. The garment should hug the hips but have a full flair at the bottom. *The heavier woman* can also wear tennis shorts of medium length rather than tennis dresses.

The long-legged woman will benefit from a short-skirted effect, and socks worn "up," to break the line of the legs

Legs too thin—you should wear medium-length tennis shorts or a tennis dress with very little flair at the bottom.

Legs too long—wear tennis socks up on leg (not folded down). This gives the illusion of a shorter leg.

Legs too short—wear tennis "half socks" or peds in tennis shoes with no socks. This will make your legs appear longer.

Any color goes on the court now, so if you are on the heavy side, wear colors instead of white. Even the darker pastels will help give you a slimmer look.

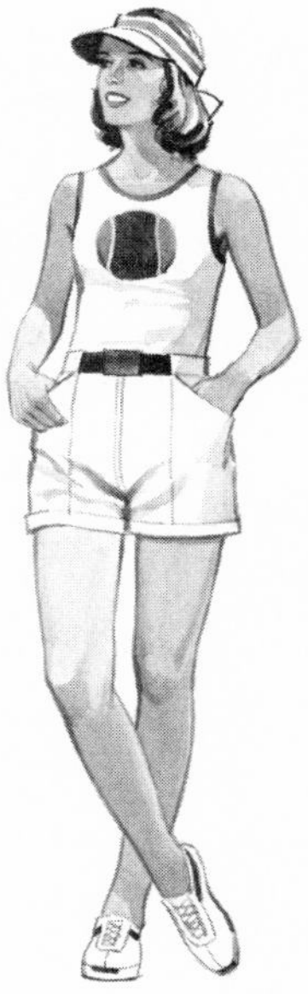

Too-short legs will benefit from short shorts and tennis half-socks or peds

GOLF WEAR

Golf skirts, culottes, Bermuda shorts, or slacks are all acceptable on the golf course. This allows a great deal of choice to women of all shapes and sizes. Golf skirts and culottes are more suited for the heavy-set woman—they soften or camouflage whatever needs to be softened or camouflaged. Sleeved shirts are better than sleeveless ones.

The woman who is too thin will look best in slacks or full (but not too full) culottes or skirts. Again, sleeved blouses will look best.

The tall woman should wear skirts (not too skimpy) or golf shorts of thin fabric with knee socks, or wear slacks.

The short woman should wear skirts, not too full, reaching just above the knee.

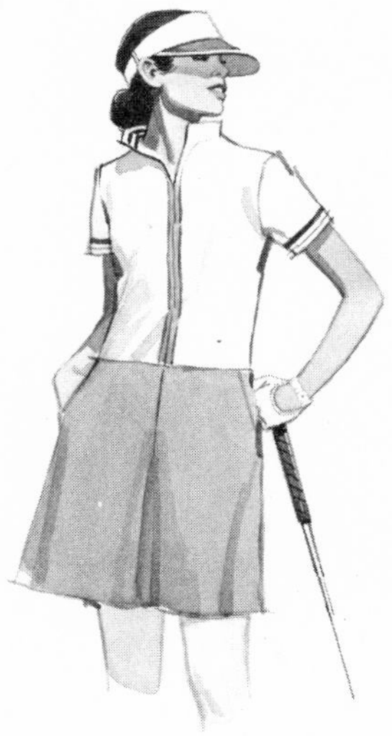

Golf skirts and culottes can slenderize the heavy-set figure

SWIM WEAR

Swimsuits are usually the article of sportswear that give women with figure problems the greatest degree of mental anguish. But there is a swimsuit style that can enable every woman to step onto the beach with confidence. There are basically three types of swimsuits: bikini, the two-piece, and the one-piece.

The bikini, in any of its variations, is only for the average to slim figure, the body in good proportion and condition. A bikini will not only fail to flatter a figure with even the slightest problems, but will actually highlight them (for example, it will cut under a full stomach and emphasize it). The string bikini in particular is only for the perfect figure, though there are styles with a little more fabric on the sides for the woman with a slightly fuller hip.

The heavy woman should wear the one-piece suit with a front panel or skirt. Keeping the lines smooth and simple avoids a bulky look. A V-neck is more slenderizing and the fabric should fall close to the hips with a flair at the bottom of the skirt. Avoid large prints and horizontal lines. Vertical designs, such as piping, are desirable; and dark colors are best. Swimsuits with built-in control are also available. With the invention of new fabrics that look like jersey and support like a girdle, shaping up for fun in the sun is easier than ever before.

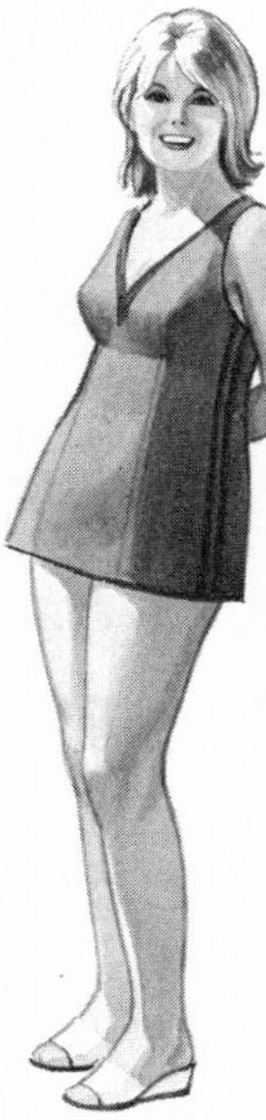

The heavy woman should wear a one-piece swimsuit

The too-thin woman should wear the type of swimsuit that has legs that look like shorts. Don't buy a skirt-type with gathers at the hem (it makes your legs look thinner). Light colors, tiny design prints, horizontal designs are best. The heavier fabrics like velour, which is soft and sensual, but thick, are good for your figure type.

The thin but not skinny woman looks best in the two-piece, with no gathers of any kind. Do not wear black or dark brown.

The too-thin (or *too-heavy*) *woman* should avoid novelty closures of any kind.

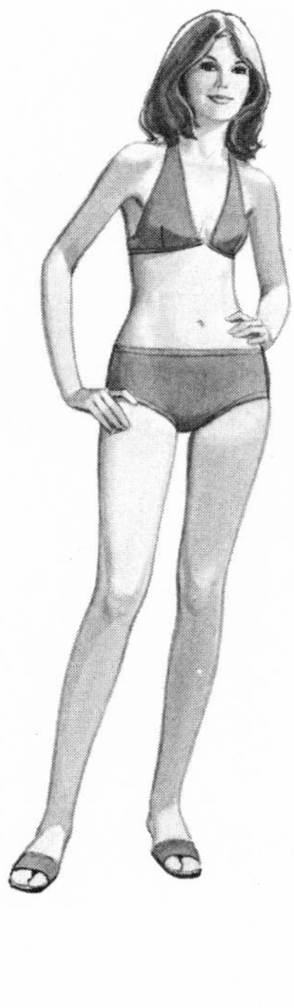

Only the slender or well-proportioned figure should wear the bikini styles

The small-busted woman can profit from gathered and shirred-top styles. The halter-top, one-piece suit is a very flattering look that will often be especially so on this figure type. There are also one- and two-piece suits available with built-in padding of various degrees. These can give a very effective illusion because the padding is an integral part of the suit, invisibly "filling out" your own fullness.

A broad-shouldered (or *wide back*) figure will profit from a shoulder-strap style, to break the expanse of shoulders and back. Swimsuits with a stripe of contrasting color down the side will usually have a slimming effect.

Swimsuit sizes go up to 38DD. If you have a body-balancing problem, a different-size top can be bought to go with a different-size bottom.

SKI WEAR

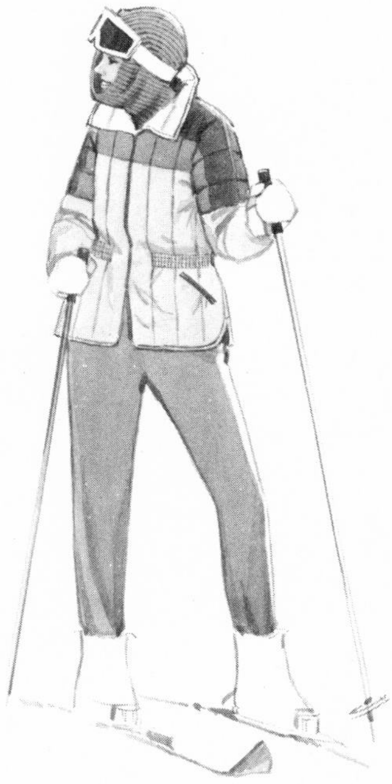

The too-thin figure can profit from bulky and heavily insulated skiwear styles

The range of styles, colors, and designs even in something so simple as a goosedown vest, is outstanding in the case of ski wear. There are options in ski clothes for every figure type. With the aid of your old friend the full-length mirror, keep trying on till you find the garment or combination of garments that you know does something special for *you*.

The heavy woman should, of course, stay away from the heavily insulated fabrics that give a bulky appearance. Stay away also from ski clothes that fit overly tight. Sometimes trying on the next size will help solve that problem. Darker-colored skiwear will give you the appearance of being slimmer. Designs should run vertical rather than horizontal.

The too-thin woman can wear the heavily insulated, bulky fabrics. Lighter colors give the illusion of added weight. If you are too tall and thin, wear a two-piece suit rather than a one-piece jumpsuit. The fun vests would also give you the illusion of added weight.

The following are some all-purpose items of sportswear, with a consideration of how they may add to (or detract from) your overall figure illusion.

WARM-UPS (also called jogging suits)

These "dashing" garments come in a wide variety of colors, usually decorated with stripes or bands. They are most commonly two-piece outfits, with long-sleeved tops and pullover pants with a zipper front.

The too-thin woman should choose lighter colors, horizontal designs, bulkier fabrics, and "front-pocket pouch" styles.

The heavy woman should choose darker colors, vertical designs (the stripe down the side of the arm and legs so common in warm-up suits is a definite advantage to the heavy woman), the thinner knits and other fabrics. Several thin stripes (down the side) give a more slenderizing effect than a single wide band. Avoid the color bands at shoulder seams.

The slim figure is flattered by the straight-leg pants style.

The heavy-legged or *the heavy figure* should look for the full or flaring leg styles.

The arms-too-long figure type can benefit from a style that has horizontal contrasting color bands on the arms, or wide-cuff style.

SWEATSHIRTS AND SWEATSUITS

Many of the same principles apply to those ever-so-comfortable ubiquitous garments. With sweatshirts it is good to remember that short sleeves and styles that tie at the waist and ankle with a drawstring will emphasize heaviness, as will overly large sweatshirts and highly bulky fabrics and designs (including "front-pocket pouches," hoods never likely to be used, and so on).

Sweatshirts are very likely to be decorated, and it is good to bear in mind that a design or decoration can most definitely influence your figure illusion. Even the lettering of a name, or large initials, can flatter or detract, depending on the individual problem—for example, a long name printed across the chest or back in large letters will create an undesirable horizontal emphasis for the heavy or broad-shouldered figure.

Remember to keep your slacks plain if your sweatshirt is "highly designed."

T-shirts are another sportswear item often appropriated for wider use. If you are too thin or too heavy, be sure to wear your T-shirt slightly loose. A T-shirt that is too tight is likely to show—all too clearly—things like bra straps and other undergarment construction details in addition to whatever flaws your figure may have.

Heavy- or thin-armed women should wear the longer styles of sleeve when possible.

Round-, heavy-, or square-faced women should wear V-necked, not high-necked styles, as should women with short necks. When wearing a drawstring style, be sure to wear one cut farther away from the face.

The too-thin woman can often profit from a leotard or a camisole worn under a T-shirt.

The same remarks made about decoration, under *Sweatshirts,* apply equally well to T's (with the added consideration that even greater care must be taken with the generally more revealing fabrics and styles of these tops).

JEANS

Jeans are an item of sportswear that can be worn many places, depending on what you wear with them and what shape they are in.

FOR CASUAL WEAR:

1. make sure they are clean and well-fitting (which means not baggy, and not overly tight—especially if you are on the heavy side)
2. patches and decorations are ok but rips and stains are not
3. if one hem is frayed, make sure both are

FOR DRESS WEAR:

1. they must be well pressed, and preferably creased front and back
2. they should have hems rather than frayed bottoms
3. they should be simply styled, rather than covered with novelty hardware, cut-outs, or tricky decorations
4. a smart blouse or shirt or jacket is needed to complete the dressy jean look
5. shoes worn with dressy jeans should be an appropriate smart daytime style

The heavy-hipped woman should wear flared-leg jeans. They are more comfortable and have a soft look that can help balance this figure type. The slim or slim-hipped woman can best wear straight-leg jeans.

The heavy-set woman should avoid jeans with a thick fold, or placket, over the zipper, bulky belt loops, and thick bulky seams. Thick materials such as corduroy and brushed denim tend to be less flattering.

The hips-too-wide type should choose styles without pockets and complex yokes.

The too-slim figure will look best in jeans with pockets and other trim.

The medium-to-slender figure and the short-waisted woman should choose hip-hugger styles.

The well-proportioned (or perfect) figure is the only one that can carry off stretch jeans.

You should be as concerned with the length of jeans as of expensive evening pants. They should be ½ inch above the bottom of the shoe, almost touching the top of the toe.

SHORTS

There are basically three types: short shorts, regular (mid-thigh length) shorts, and Bermuda shorts. Needless to say, only a young woman with great legs should wear short shorts.

Regular shorts can be worn by those who are not overweight or only slightly overweight.

If your legs are heavy (if you are heavy in general), or if your legs are too thin, wear Bermuda shorts (which extend to the lower thigh or just above the knee).

Short shorts—the shorter, the better, within reason—can help a short-legged woman appear longer legged (and the slash-side style or slant-leg is even better than cuffed styles for this purpose). Remember that too much decoration (pockets, trim, and so on) can make hips look heavy even if they are not. And the micro-short shorts are too likely to show undergarments and other things better concealed when you move or bend, to be really desirable for any figure type to wear in public.

SOCKS

Though socks of many kinds serve a wide variety of sportswear functions, they seem to be less flattering to the leg than, say, stockings (which have been discussed in other chapters). Socks, especially cuffed socks, have a tendency to "cut off" the leg and create a stubby look; they also, unfortunately, exaggerate the problem of large feet.

Socks are an accessory that can easily be overdone (colors, patterns, decorations, tassels, etc.) unless you happen to be a teenager.

The heavy-legged woman should avoid bulky high socks, and socks with cuffs. If socks are necessary, then wear the thinnest type available, with a vertical weave if possible.

The thin-legged woman can wear bulky, high socks beneath Bermuda shorts or a tennis dress to give the look of heavier legs.

In general, light colors and patterns of any kind will add weight to a leg. Dark and medium-dark tones will create a slimmer effect (and should therefore be avoided by the thin-legged person).

Chapter Ten

AND YOU WITH THE GREAT FIGURE

Many women with great figures give the illusion of *not* having one. This is mostly due to carelessness, as shown by wrong choice of clothes: accessories, fabric, and design. A good study in a full-length mirror would help to correct this. But remember that all four views must be studied: back, front, and both sides.

Many women with basically good figures spoil the illusion by overdoing it—putting too many colors, too many designs, too much jewelry together. Remember: *Keep it simple.* Let your figure speak for, and by, itself.

The following are examples of oversight and carelessness that can detract from even the greatest of figures:

1. Wearing something—anything—that doesn't fit properly. If it doesn't fit, get it fitted or learn to do it yourself. If you are wearing a belt because a garment waistline is too big, sew the waist up and get the proper fit.
2. Pinning things together. If you're in a pinned-together state as you're reading this, stop right now and sew.
3. Wearing too many accessories together, too much eye-catching trim—a scarf around the neck with a necklace; a pendant with bracelets and rings; chains and discs on handbags, belts and shoes—all this is ruinous to a good appearance. Remember: *keep it simple.*
4. Mixing dressy items with sporty ones, faddy casual items with elegant ones. Examples would be a dressy turban with a casual outfit; clunky shoes with a delicate evening bag; daytime accessories (shoes, jewelry, scarves) mixed with dressy clothes; or dressy shoes to the office.
5. Hanging, uneven, or poorly executed hems.
6. Pants length too short or too long. Pants should touch the top of the toe of the shoe in front and be ½ inch from the floor in back.

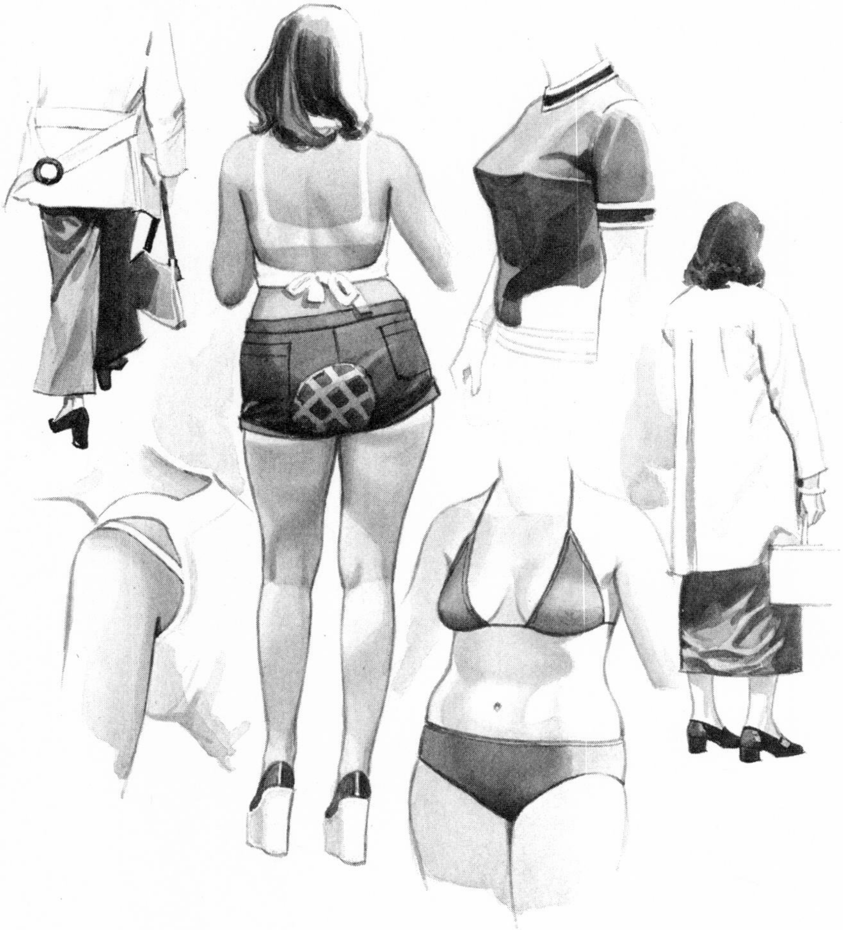

7. Wrinkled or unpressed garments.
8. Slip or bra straps showing.
9. Stains or spots on clothing.
10. Missing buttons.
11. Pulls in knits, hanging threads.
12. Tears in clothing, split seams.
13. Lint or hairs on dark-colored clothes.
14. Soiled bra or slip straps, collars and cuffs, stained underarms.
15. Baggy stockings.
16. Runs in stockings or panty-hose. (For special occasions, always carry an extra pair in a plastic bag in your handbag.)

17. Oversized platform shoes.
18. Light shoes with dark skirt, dress, or pants (see Chapter Eight).
19. Run-down shoes. Keep shoes resoled and reheeled.
20. Suntan lines that contrast dramatically with the garment you have on.
21. An ill-fitting bra "cutting into" the body beneath a form-fitting top.
22. Underpants "line" showing through slacks. This is not sexy, it's sloppy (see Chapter Seven).
23. Overly tight garments.
24. Outdated and unflattering styles.

INDEX